Value-Added Electrodiagnostics

Editors

KAREN P. BARR
ILEANA M. HOWARD

PHYSICAL MEDICINE AND REHABILITATION CLINICS OF NORTH AMERICA

www.pmr.theclinics.com

Consulting Editor
SANTOS F. MARTINEZ

November 2018 • Volume 29 • Number 4

ELSEVIER

1600 John F. Kennedy Boulevard • Suite 1800 • Philadelphia, Pennsylvania, 19103-2899

http://www.theclinics.com

PHYSICAL MEDICINE AND REHABILITATION CLINICS OF NORTH AMERICA Volume 29, Number 4
November 2018 ISSN 1047-9651, ISBN 978-0-323-64153-1

Editor: Lauren Boyle
Developmental Editor: Meredith Madeira

Reprints. For copies of 100 or more of articles in this publication, please contact the Commercial Reprints Department, Elsevier Inc., 360 Park Avenue South, New York, NY 10010-1710. Tel.: 212-633-3874; Fax: 212-633-3820; E-mail: reprints@elsevier.com.

Physical Medicine and Rehabilitation Clinics of North America (ISSN 1047-9651) is published quarterly by Elsevier Inc., 360 Park Avenue South, New York, NY 10010-1710. Months of issue are February, May, August, and November. Business and Editorial Offices: 1600 John F. Kennedy Blvd., Suite 1800, Philadelphia, PA 19103-2899. Customer Service Office: 3251 Riverport Lane, Maryland Heights, MO 63043. Periodicals postage paid at New York, NY and additional mailing offices. Subscription price per year is $294.00 (US individuals), $571.00 (US institutions), $100.00 (US students), $351.00 (Canadian individuals), $752.00 (Canadian institutions), $210.00 (Canadian students), $427.00 (foreign individuals), $752.00 (foreign institutions), and $210.00 (foreign students). Foreign air speed delivery is included in all *Clinics* subscription prices. All prices are subject to change without notice. **POSTMASTER:** Send address changes to *Physical Medicine and Rehabilitation Clinics of North America*, Customer Service Office: Elsevier Health Sciences Division, Subscription Customer Service, 3251 Riverport Lane, Maryland Heights, MO 63043. **Customer Service: 1-800-654-2452 (US). From outside of the United States, call 314-447-8871. Fax: 314-447-8029. E-mail: JournalsCustomer Service-usa@elsevier.com (for print support); JournalsOnlineSupport-usa@elsevier.com (for online support).**

Physical Medicine and Rehabilitation Clinics of North America is indexed in *Excerpta Medica, MEDLINE/ PubMed (Index Medicus), Cinahl,* and *Cumulative Index to Nursing and Allied Health Literature.*

Contributors

CONSULTING EDITOR

SANTOS F. MARTINEZ, MD, MS
Diplomate of the American Academy of Physical Medicine and Rehabilitation, Certificate of Added Qualification Sports Medicine, Assistant Professor, Department of Orthopaedics, Campbell Clinic Orthopaedics, The University of Tennessee, Memphis, Tennessee, USA

EDITORS

KAREN P. BARR, MD
Associate Professor, Department of Orthopaedics, Chief, Division of Physical Medicine and Rehabilitation, West Virginia University, Morgantown, West Virginia, USA

ILEANA M. HOWARD, MD
Outpatient Medical Director, Rehabilitation Care Medicine, VA Puget Sound Health Care System, Clinical Associate Professor, Department of Rehabilitation Medicine, University of Washington, Seattle, Washington, USA

AUTHORS

MICHELE L. ARNOLD, MD, FAAPMR, FAANEM
Executive Medical Director, Chief, Physical Medicine and Rehabilitation, Swedish Health Services, Seattle, Washington, USA

KAREN P. BARR, MD
Associate Professor, Department of Orthopaedics, Chief, Division of Physical Medicine and Rehabilitation, West Virginia University, Morgantown, West Virginia, USA

KEVIN BARRETTE, MD
Department of Orthopedics, Stanford University, Redwood City, California, USA

AARON E. BUNNELL, MD
Assistant Professor, Department of Rehabilitation Medicine, University of Washington, Seattle, Washington, USA

MEGAN CLARK, MD
Medical Director, Oncology Rehabilitation, University of Kansas, Comprehensive Spine Center, Kansas City, Kansas, USA

DAVID DEL TORO, MD
Professor, Department of Physical Medicine and Rehabilitation, Medical College of Wisconsin, Milwaukee, Wisconsin, USA

ANDREW DUBIN, MD, MS
Professor, Interim Chair, Department of Physical Medicine and Rehabilitation, Albany Medical College, Albany, New York, USA

ELBA GERENA-MALDONADO, MD
Department of Physical Medicine and Rehabilitation, Providence St. Joseph Health, Providence Medical Group, Missoula, Montana, USA

SANDRA L. HEARN, MD
Clinical Instructor, Department of Physical Medicine and Rehabilitation, Michigan Medicine, Burlington Office Center, Ann Arbor, Michigan, USA

ILEANA M. HOWARD, MD
Outpatient Medical Director, Rehabilitation Care Medicine, VA Puget Sound Health Care System, Clinical Associate Professor, Department of Rehabilitation Medicine, University of Washington, Seattle, Washington, USA

DENNIS S. KAO, MD
Assistant Professor, Department of Plastic Surgery, University of Washington, Seattle, Washington, USA

DAVID J. KENNEDY, MD
Professor, Chair, Department of Physical Medicine and Rehabilitation, Vanderbilt University Medical Center, Nashville, Tennessee, USA

JOSHUA LEVIN, MD
Department of Orthopedics and Neurosurgery, Stanford University, Palo Alto, California, USA

DEREK MILES, DPT
Department of Rehabilitation, Stanford Children's Hospital, Palo Alto, California, USA

P. ANDREW NELSON, MD
Associate Professor, Department of Physical Medicine and Rehabilitation, Medical College of Wisconsin, Milwaukee, Wisconsin, USA

NASSIM RAD, MD
Acting Assistant Professor, Department of Rehabilitation Medicine, University of Washington, Seattle, Washington, USA

JAMES K. RICHARDSON, MD
Professor, Department of Physical Medicine and Rehabilitation, Michigan Medicine, Burlington Office Center, Ann Arbor, Michigan, USA

LAWRENCE R. ROBINSON, MD
Professor, Physical Medicine and Rehabilitation, University of Toronto, Sunnybrook Health Sciences Centre, Toronto, Ontario, Canada

LEILEI WANG, MD, PhD
Clinical Associate Professor, Department of Rehabilitation Medicine, School of Medicine, University of Washington, Seattle, Washington, USA

Contents

Walking confers numerous health benefits, particularly for middle-aged and older patients with diabetes and metabolic syndrome. Nevertheless, it brings a risk of injurious falls, especially among populations with diabetes and metabolic syndrome–related distal neuromuscular decline and frank neuropathy. Those who stand to benefit most from walking are at greatest risk. Development of practical clinical tools to more precisely quantify neuromuscular function and link it to mobility outcomes will help clinicians target interventions toward those at risk for falls. Electrodiagnosis, with inclusion of several newer techniques, serves as a promising tool for objective evaluation of distal neuromuscular function.

This article provides physiatrists, neurologists, and neuromuscular medicine physicians a framework that can be easily used in the process of evaluating, identifying, and treating patients with toxic myopathies. This article attempts to classify these rare but potentially deadly conditions in clinical patterns and distinguishes the cellular mechanisms in which the offending agents tend to affect the structure and function of myocytes.

Electrodiagnostic testing provides insight into subclinical aspects of disease in amyotrophic lateral sclerosis and helps one to diagnose and exclude other diagnoses. It may also help in managing or tracking disease progression. Mapping the extent of subclinical disease may guide the clinician to supportive interventions. There is considerable interest in establishing electrodiagnostic biomarkers to monitor disease progression. This article details the usefulness of electrodiagnostic testing across the disease spectrum. A review of clinical presentations and differential diagnoses, diagnostic evaluation, and emerging applications of electrodiagnostic studies to guide management and assess response to treatment interventions are presented with considerations for clinical practice.

In the electrodiagnostic (EDX) approach of the patient who presents with foot pain, numbness, and/or tingling, it is important to consider a broad differential diagnosis of both neuropathic and nonneuropathic conditions, including focal and systemic causes. This article assists the electromyographer in the selection and utilization of the most appropriate EDX studies for evaluation. The EDX findings and impression can then help guide potential treatment options for the patient with foot pain and other symptoms. Moreover, this discussion demonstrates the added value that EDX evaluation of the foot provides to the comprehensive assessment of foot pain.

PHYSICAL MEDICINE AND REHABILITATION CLINICS OF NORTH AMERICA

SERIES OF RELATED INTEREST

Orthopedic Clinics
Clinics in Sports Medicine
Neurologic Clinics

VISIT THE CLINICS ONLINE!
Access your subscription at:
www.theclinics.com

Foreword

Taking Electrodiagnostics a Step Further

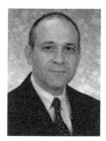

Santos F. Martinez, MD, MS
Consulting Editor

Electrodiagnostics has been an integral component of the basic physical medicine and rehabilitation curriculum for decades. Most of our residency programs require completion of a minimum number of studies to sit for board examination. This branch of our training allows further appreciation and objective documentation of a wide field of neuropathic and myopathic conditions. Dynamic electromyography also extends to other disciplines by providing ancillary functional and kinesiologic/biomechanical data, whether it be for clarifying neurologic conditions or for delineating task-oriented recruitment patterns for performance optimization.

This issue of the *Physical Medicine and Rehabilitation Clinics of North America* does not follow the typical electrodiagnostic format. Dr Barr and Dr Howard have turned what could be a very mundane topic into a clinically relevant and dynamic issue. They extend upon the readers' basic foundation of physical medicine and rehabilitation and evolve from basic data interpretation to guidance in patient management. This certainly will impact not only our patients directly but also possibly those physicians who are seeking treatment and prognostic clues from our consultative interpretations. I thank the Guest Editors and authors for their foresight and ingenuity in developing this issue.

Santos F. Martinez, MD, MS
American Academy of Physical
Medicine and Rehabilitation
Campbell Clinic Orthopaedics
Department of Orthopaedics
University of Tennessee
Memphis, TN 38104, USA

E-mail address:
smartinez@campbellclinic.com

Phys Med Rehabil Clin N Am 29 (2018) xi
https://doi.org/10.1016/j.pmr.2018.07.002
1047-9651/18/© 2018 Published by Elsevier Inc.

Preface

The Value Electrodiagnosis Adds to Patient Care: Making It Transparent

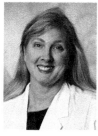 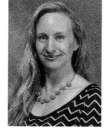

Karen P. Barr, MD   Ileana M. Howard, MD
Editors

A focus on value in health care has been described by thought leaders as the "strategy that will fix health care," with achieving high value for the patient as "the overarching goal of health care delivery." Yet, this term is also used as a code word for cost reduction by reducing services, rather than as a framework for performance improvement.[1,2] There is a risk that without our collective voices being heard, the value of electrodiagnosis will be underrecognized and much will be lost in the name of cost containment.

The editors and authors in this issue have spent their medical careers performing electrodiagnostic consultations that not only provide diagnostic clarity but also add value to patient care; not only by the localization of peripheral nerve lesions or the identification of muscle disease but also by providing information that guides treatment decisions, informs patients about their prognosis, and helps prevent serious disability by identifying patients at high risk for falls, diabetes, and other potentially life-threatening conditions.

The purpose of this issue is to make this value transparent to our readers. Our expert authors discuss the value that electrodiagnosis adds to a multitude of diagnoses, from carpal tunnel syndrome to foot pain; from sudden onset traumatic injuries to slowly progressive systemic diseases. We hope that it is helpful for electrodiagnosticians who want to design and perform the most current, evidence-based studies, for other health care providers to understand how best to utilize electrodiagnosis in the care of

Phys Med Rehabil Clin N Am 29 (2018) xiii–xiv
https://doi.org/10.1016/j.pmr.2018.07.001
1047-9651/18/© 2018 Published by Elsevier Inc.

their patients, and for policymakers, payers, and health care system leaders to better understand the value electrodiagnosis provides.

Karen P. Barr, MD
Department of Orthopaedics
Division of PM&R
West Virginia University
1 Medical Center Drive
Box 9100
Morgantown, WV 26506, USA

Ileana M. Howard, MD
Department of Rehabilitation Medicine
University of Washington
S-117 RCS
1660 South Columbian Way
Seattle, WA 98108, USA

E-mail addresses:
karen.barr@hsc.wvu.edu (K.P. Barr)
ileana.howard@va.gov (I.M. Howard)

REFERENCES

1. Porter ME. What is value in health care? N Engl J Med 2010;363(26):2477–81.
2. Porter ME, Lee TH. The strategy that will fix health care. Harvard Business Review 2013.

Value-Added Electrodiagnostics

Targeting Interventions for Fall Risk Reduction

Sandra L. Hearn, MD*, James K. Richardson, MD

KEYWORDS

- Neuropathy • Falls • Walking • Neuromuscular decline • Nerve conduction studies
- Electromyography • Medial plantar • Electrodiagnosis

KEY POINTS

- Walking and exercise confer important health benefits, but these benefits are threatened by the risk of injurious falls.
- Distal neuromuscular ability represents a continuum of function; thus, detection of early or subclinical neuromuscular decline can inform fall risk.
- Electrodiagnosis holds promise as an objective measure of distal neuromuscular function. The medial plantar sensory nerve conduction study, electromyography of distal foot muscles, and interpretation of fibular motor amplitudes on a functional basis may increase sensitivity for detection of early, yet functionally relevant, distal neuromuscular decline.
- Identifying patients at risk for falls enables targeting of interventions to reduce fall risk and allow patients to walk and exercise safely.

THERE IS A NEED TO IDENTIFY PATIENTS AT RISK FOR FALLS

The routine act of walking confers many health benefits and represents a vitally important activity throughout the human lifespan. Walking is associated with decreased mortality in men[1] and decreased coronary events[2] and cognitive decline[3] in women. Among those with type 2 diabetes mellitus, it slows decline in mobility,[4] improves glycemic control,[5] and is associated with lower total mortality.[6] These findings should beckon health care providers to recommend walking and routine exercise for their patients for as long as safely possible.

Unfortunately, in older adults with declining neuromuscular function, walking comes with the increased risk of falling. In fact, patient populations with arguably the greatest

Disclosure Statement: No disclosures (S.L. Hearn). This work was supported by the National Institutes of Health ROI 5R01 AG026569 (J.K. Richardson).
Department of Physical Medicine and Rehabilitation, Michigan Medicine, 325 E Eisenhower Parkway Suite 100, Ann Arbor, MI 48108-3364, USA
* Corresponding author.
E-mail address: slhearn@med.umich.edu

need for the therapeutic effects of walking harbor greater risk of falling. Neuropathy is a well-established risk factor for falls,[7] and it is associated with type 2 diabetes mellitus as well as the metabolic syndrome[8,9]—both conditions for which walking and exercise are recommended. Without exercise, a vicious cycle ensues, in which diminished peripheral nerve function can lead to diminished activity, which may, in turn, raise risk factors for neuropathy (**Fig. 1**). The risk of falls thus poses a quandary for clinicians: although walking confers many health advantages, the increased risk of injurious falls in the very populations that stand to benefit undercuts its advantages. There is a need to guide recommendations based on quantifiable physiologic risk factors for falls during ambulation. In particular, an ability to predict who, among patients, is likely to fall, would enable targeting of interventions to prevent falls, and empower clinicians to appropriately and confidently guide patients to maximize safe walking and improve their function and health.

DISTAL NEUROMUSCULAR IMPAIRMENT CONTRIBUTES TOWARD FALLS RISK

Recent research has advanced the understanding of why we fall. In particular, falls tend to occur during ambulation on uneven or irregular surfaces[10] where an unexpected perturbation in balance requires the patient to make a corrective step within a sufficient timeframe to prevent a fall. From this process follow 2 major categories for falls risk factors: neuromuscular and neurocognitive attributes.

The seminal work of Lord and colleagues[11] identified 5 physiologic fall risk factors, with 3 of them (knee flexion repositioning maneuver, knee extensor strength, and standing sway) associated with lower limb neuromuscular function. The authors have worked to organize these critical neuromuscular attributes into a conceptual model that links neuromuscular and neurocognitive elements essential for maintaining balance when encountering unexpected perturbations during ambulation[12] (**Fig. 2**).

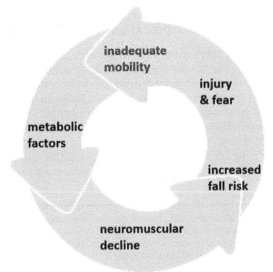

Fig. 1. Without exercise, a vicious cycle ensues, in which metabolic risk factors lead to diminished peripheral nerve function, which in turn, diminishes activity. This figure was created using graphics available on openclipart.com; the component graphics are available under the Creative Commons Zero 1.0 Public Domain License.

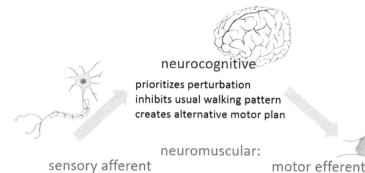

neurocognitive

prioritizes perturbation
inhibits usual walking pattern
creates alternative motor plan

neuromuscular:

sensory afferent   motor efferent
relays perturbation   executes motor plan

Fig. 2. Components of afferent sensory, neurocognitive, and motor efferent aspects work together to permit a response to perturbation that averts a fall. This figure was created using openclipart.com and is available under the Creative Commons Zero 1.0 Public Domain License.

Specifically, there is need for adequate distal sensory function to quickly and precisely detect a perturbation and relay it to cognitive centers. In addition, the efferent motor pathways of nerve and muscle must rapidly generate force in key muscle groups needed to execute a corrective measure, such as a shift in center of mass or a corrective step. Although perturbation responses occurring in less than 150 milliseconds are likely subcortical in nature, responses occurring after 200 milliseconds are optimized by cortical input.[13] Given robust evidence that inhibitory executive functions are critical to gait and maintenance of balance,[14] the authors hypothesize that this neurocognitive component links the afferent and efferent components by prioritizing the afferent perturbation signal and rapidly inhibiting the default ambulatory pattern, which allows execution of an alternative motor plan (**Fig. 3**).

In support of the neuromuscular aspects of this model, the authors have developed a composite measure of ankle proprioceptive threshold (representing afferent function) and hip strength (representing efferent function) that has been shown to predict sagittal plane response to perturbation, as well as prospectively recorded falls and fall-related injuries.[15] The hip strength/ankle proprioceptive precision model also strongly predicted unipedal stance time ($R^2 = .754$) and, in so doing, rendered age insignificant as a predictor. This finding suggests that age-related decrements in hip strength and foot/ankle proprioceptive precision may, at least in part, explain the decline in unipedal stance time that is observed with age and frequently regarded as normal.

Within this model, distal peripheral nerve function emerges as an important measure of falls risk, predominantly by way of the sensory afferent pathway. Indeed, a systematic review of 8 studies has concluded that poor sensory and motor peripheral nerve function predict poor physical function and mobility disability.[16] Those with better physical function are also able to do more; a longitudinal cohort study of more than 300 subjects demonstrated that peripheral nerve function is modestly positively associated with self-reported activity as well as vigorous physical activity among older men.[17] Of particular importance, the relationship between neuromuscular function and mobility outcomes is continuous, such that more severe neuropathy scores are associated with poorer mobility outcomes. Given the nature of this relationship, one should seek measures that can assess degree of distal neuromuscular impairment, and not merely the presence or absence of a disease, such as neuropathy.

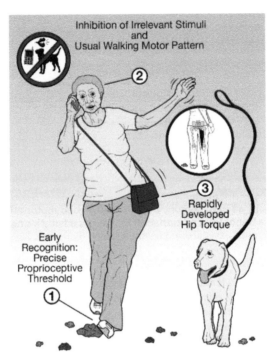

Fig. 3. The proposed sequence of neuromuscular and cognitive events required for successful response to perturbation while walking. The woman depicted has 400 to 500 milliseconds to alter right foot placement after encountering the perturbation with the left foot. In that interval, she must: (1) recognize the perturbation; (2) inhibit irrelevant afferent stimuli and inhibit the preplanned step; (3) generate sufficient torque in key stance and swing limb muscles to adjust right foot placement. (*Adapted from* Richardson JK. Imbalanced: The confusing, circular nature of falls research... and a possible antidote. Am J Phys Med Rehab 2017;96(1):55; with permission.)

Where clinical measures of distal neuromuscular function fall short due to reliance on patient attention, effort, or relaxation, electrodiagnostic measures offer objective information and routinely record from the distal lower limb. Electrodiagnosticians are poised to objectively evaluate neuromuscular function, including that which impacts mobility and fall risk but falls short of unequivocal neuropathy.

NEUROMUSCULAR DECLINE OCCURS ON A CONTINUUM AND INFLUENCES FALL RISK

Epidemiologic, radiologic, and electrophysiologic studies indicate that neuromuscular decline occurs along a continuum. As a result, there is a corresponding decline from optimal mobility function, which precedes clinical diagnosis of neuropathy. Longitudinal data from more than 900 individuals with diabetic neuropathy and matched controls over 14 years show that among older adults, those with neuropathy are a greater risk for falls, and that their rate of falling increases over time.[18] Of particular relevance to this discussion, the increase in fall risk can be detected as early as 3 to 5 years before diagnosis of peripheral neuropathy, underscoring that functionally relevant decline in neuromuscular function precedes diagnosis of neuropathy.

Imaging of distal foot muscles parallels the clinical observation of early neuromuscular decline, revealing that progressive distal muscular atrophy occurs early in the course of disease. Patients with diabetic neuropathy were found to have a reduction in intrinsic foot muscle volume of about 50% compared with matched controls.[19] Patients with diabetes but without neuropathy did not manifest this loss. A cohort of 26 patients with type 1 diabetes mellitus showed 3.0% decline in foot muscle volume per year, compared with 1.1% in nonneuropathic patients and 0.2% for controls.[20] The loss in muscle mass was associated with neuropathy severity; over the course of 13 years, muscle volume in the lower leg diminished by greater than 50% among those with severe neuropathy, whereas those with milder neuropathy lost about 20% of foot muscle volume. The clinical relevance of these findings is brought out by biomechanical research identifying foot intrinsic muscles as significant contributors to medial-lateral stability during unipedal stance.[21]

Finally, electrodiagnostic measures of neuromuscular decline also predict function. In a prospective cohort study of greater than 2000 subjects, low fibular motor amplitude (defined as <1 mV) predicted mobility disability over the course of a median of 8.5 years.[22] Through laboratory-based work, the authors have independently demonstrated that fibular motor amplitude predicts distal sensory and motor function as well as fall risk (detailed in the following section). Taken together, the epidemiologic, radiological, and electrodiagnostic findings presented above reinforce that neuropathy is not simply a binary clinical entity or risk factor for falls, to be evaluated as present or absent. Rather, neuropathy entails a process of gradual distal neuromuscular decline that occurs along a continuum with functional relevance, clearly preceding a clinical diagnosis of neuropathy. It follows that prompt detection of this early decline in neuromuscular status may offer early identification of those individuals at risk for falls, regardless of whether they meet current clinical or electrodiagnostic criteria for axonal peripheral polyneuropathy.

MECHANISMS BY WHICH DECLINING NEUROMUSCULAR FUNCTION CAN INFLUENCE MOBILITY AND FALL RISK

The authors' laboratory-based work relating fibular motor amplitudes to ankle frontal plane motor and sensory function offers a plausible mechanism by which decrements in peripheral neuromuscular function may influence mobility and fall risk. The authors studied older subjects with a spectrum of peripheral nerve function, ranging from moderate diabetic neuropathy to healthy and quantified their frontal plane sensory and motor ankle functions. To quantify sensory function, they used a specially designed cradle apparatus that allowed the determination of inversion/eversion proprioceptive thresholds while the subject was weight-bearing (**Fig. 4**). Motor function was evaluated with subjects standing on a force plate; during ankle inversion maneuvers, the speed of translation of the ground reaction force was measured. Electrodiagnostic testing was performed with Carefusion Nicolet electromyographs with Viking 4 Software.

The authors found that electrodiagnostic data predicted both the sensory and the motor measures of function. Fibular motor amplitudes recording at the extensor digitorum brevis strongly correlated with frontal plane (inversion/eversion) ankle proprioceptive precision (**Fig. 5**A) as well as with rate of ankle inversion torque generation (**Fig. 5**B)—both factors that influence postural stability and recovery from perturbation during gait.[23] In the authors' sample of older subjects with a spectrum of peripheral neurologic function, the fibular motor amplitude predicted almost 60% of proprioceptive threshold. Importantly, this relationship persisted when subjects with neuropathy, as evidenced by fibular motor amplitudes less than 2.0 mV, were excluded. Therefore, among the ostensibly "normal" subjects, correlation between ankle proprioception and fibular motor amplitude was robust (**Fig. 5**A). This finding reinforces that functionally relevant declines in neuromuscular function occur well before clinical neuropathy

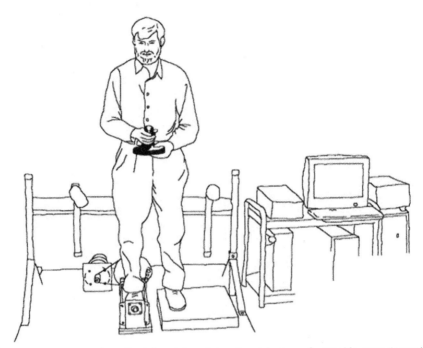

Fig. 4. Apparatus and method for determining frontal plane foot/ankle proprioceptive thresholds. Eighty suprathreshold and infrathreshold inverting and everting stimuli, interspersed with 20 "dummy" trials associated with no cradle motion, were presented sequentially using a psychometrically valid double-staircase technique. The subject moved the joystick in the direction of perceived motion or held it in midline if no motion was suspected. A proprioceptive threshold, in degrees, at which the subject was 100% accurate was derived. Note that a smaller proprioceptive threshold is more precise, or "better." (*From* Richardson JK, Allet L, Kim H, et al. Fibular motor nerve conduction studies and ankle sensorimotor capacities. Muscle Nerve 2013;47(4):499; with permission.)

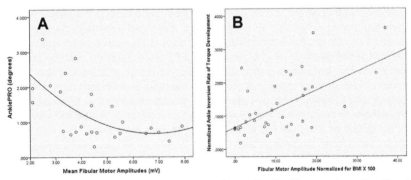

Fig. 5. (*A*) The relationship between laboratory-determined ankle proprioceptive threshold and fibular motor amplitude in a group of 26 older subjects without neuropathy. Only those with fibular motor amplitude greater than 2.0 mV (above the lower limit of normal per laboratory-specific cutoff) are included. The data were best fit with a quadratic model ($R^2 = 0.386$), suggesting that fibular motor amplitude greater than approximately 4.0 mV predicts optimal proprioceptive precision. (*B*) Fibular motor amplitude predicts normalized ankle inversion rate of torque development in a group of 37 older subjects with and without neuropathy ($R^2 = 0.364$). BMI, body mass index.

is diagnosed, and that the decline is electrodiagnostically quantifiable. That this single electrodiagnostic parameter predicted both sensory function as well as conjoined fibular and tibial-mediated motor function (ankle inversion) (**Fig. 5**B) suggests that it can serve as a measure of general distal nerve function. Finally, and perhaps of greatest relevance, fibular motor amplitude, when combined with lateral plank time as a clinical estimate of hip strength,[24] prospectively predicted falls over 1 year (**Table 1**). The robust predictive value (effect size 2.3) of fibular motor amplitude multiplied by 5 and combined with lateral plank time prompts consideration of whether a simple measure of lateral plank time, obtained readily in the electrodiagnostic laboratory and interpreted in conjunction with the fibular motor amplitude, could enable meaningful quantification of fall risk. The emerging understanding of how neuromuscular decline informs fall risk invites expansion of the traditional use of electrodiagnosis—beyond disease definition and into a tool that informs clinicians regarding clinically relevant function and risk.

ELECTRODIAGNOSIS CAN OBJECTIVELY DETECT EARLY DISTAL NEUROMUSCULAR DECLINE

Given the apparent functional relevance of early neuromuscular decline, it would behoove electrodiagnosticians to develop ways to detect it. Nevertheless, the electrodiagnostic literature concerning peripheral neuromuscular dysfunction has largely focused on markers that appear to harbor only modest sensitivity for early neuropathy. The minimum case definition for axonal neuropathy is an abnormality (99th or first percentile) of any attribute of nerve conduction in 2 separate nerves, one of which must be the sural nerve.[25] Electrodiagnostic criteria for axonal neuropathy are not met if the fibular motor and sural studies are both normal. Because these criteria rely on population normative data, they identify, by definition, only the lowest 1% of the population without an overt neuropathy phenotype. However, estimates of the sensitivity of the sural sensory amplitude for detecting neuropathy range from only 29% to 62%,[26] suggesting that the current electrodiagnostic criteria often fail to detect early neuropathy, in addition to clinically relevant distal neuromuscular decline. In fact, electrodiagnosticians have responded to the apparent age-related neuromuscular decline by downshifting the normative thresholds and adjusting for age. Although it remains unclear whether these earlier and milder phenotypes should represent a disease entity, such as early neuropathy, or whether they would be better classified along the spectrum of age-related neuromuscular decline, the continuous relationship between neuromuscular decline and mobility outcomes argues that these phenotypes are functionally relevant and likely predict falls risk. There is a need to better develop and attend to objective electrodiagnostic markers of early distal neuromuscular decline with functional relevance.

Table 1
Lateral plank time and fibular motor amplitude serve as clinical estimates of laboratory-based measures of hip strength and ankle proprioceptive precision, respectively, which are strongly associated with falls and unipedal stance time

	No Fall	+ Fall	P Value	Effect Size
Lateral Plank Time (seconds)	23 ± 10	9.3 ± 8.8	<.001	1.5
F M Amp (mV)	5.3 ± 1.4	2.2 ± 2.1	<.001	1.7
LPT + F M Amp × 5	48 ± 12	19 ± 14	<.001	2.3

Note that fibular motor amplitude (F M Amp) (multiplied by 5 to achieve similar magnitude as lateral plank time [LPT]) and added to LPT demonstrated a robust effect size of 2.3.

Potential reasons for the limited sensitivity of standard nerve conduction studies in the detection of early distal neuromuscular decline include the following:

- Standard nerve conduction studies fail to record the most distal regions of the body, which are known to be affected earliest in a length-dependent process. Specifically, the sural sensory study records from the proximal lateral foot and does not relay information about nerve fibers at the level of the forefoot or toes.
- Because normal responses show broad variance across the population, with the lower limit of normal declining with age (based on normative data adjusted for age-related neuromuscular decline), a significant amount of axon loss can be required to meet criteria for abnormality. As an example, the authors' laboratory normative range for the sural sensory response amplitude can range from 4 μV to 35 μV for patients older than 60 years of age, implying that an individual with a sural response of 20 μV can develop neuropathy, lose 75% of recordable sural nerve axons so as to exhibit a sural sensory amplitude of 5 μV, and still be considered normal. Furthermore, many laboratories consider an absent sural response within normal limits in individuals beyond the age of 70 years.[27] In this regard, using the electrodiagnostic definition of neuropathy above, early neuropathy cannot be confirmed in subjects older than 70 years of age.
- Nerve conduction studies underestimate axon loss in slow, chronic processes because amplitudes can recover in the setting of reinnervation.
- Because the great majority of electrodiagnostic studies represent initial studies of the limb, the data obtained fail to inform about the trajectory of the patient's neuromuscular status. How the rate of neuromuscular decline influences function remains unclear; perhaps a more rapid decline carries a greater impact on function, as the central nervous system grapples with the rapidly changing afferent information.

Fortunately, recent research has brought electrodiagnostic techniques that hold promise for increased sensitivity for early distal neuromuscular decline. First, study of the medial plantar nerve permits more distal sampling, increasing sensitivity in a length-dependent process. Second, needle electromyography of a distal foot muscle offers distal anatomic representation as well as the known sensitivity of electromyography for even small amounts of axon loss. Finally, the routine fibular motor amplitude recorded from the extensor digitorum brevis muscle can be interpreted from a functional, rather than diagnostic, perspective, as described in the previous section. The authors detail these approaches in later discussion.

Mixed Medial Plantar Studies

Study of the medial plantar nerves offers a more distal exploration for a length-dependent process, which would plausibly increase sensitivity. Studies to date have shown that the medial plantar nerve conduction technique demonstrates good intra-observer and interobserver reproducibility[28] and that the response can be reliably obtained in subjects younger than 70 years of age, although amplitudes can be low (one study suggests 2 μV in the sixth decade and 1 μV in the seventh decade of age as lower limits of normal).[29] Three studies independently showed that the medial plantar response significantly improves sensitivity for neuropathy in cases with clinical evidence of distal symmetric polyneuropathy, with reported sensitivities of 69% (compared with 27% for the sural study),[29] 91% (compared with 55% for the sural study),[30] and 59% (compared with 24% for the sural study)[28] with specificity held at >95% or 2 standard deviations of normal. Two additional studies found a sensitivity of 42.9% (among those with clinical symptoms of large-fiber neuropathy)[31] and 60%

(among those with clinical diabetic neuropathy)[32] in patient populations with normal sural nerve conduction studies. Finally, the medial plantar response amplitude correlates with severity of neuropathy as measured clinically by the Diabetic Neuropathy Symptom scale, adding support for its reflection of a disease process.[33] In the authors' laboratory, medial plantar sensory studies are frequently obtained in patients with a clinical presentation consistent with neuropathy in whom sural nerve conduction responses exhibit normal or borderline amplitudes.

Electromyography of a Distal Dorsal Foot Muscle

Electromyography of a distal foot muscle appeals as a method for detecting early distal neuromuscular decline for 2 reasons: it offers distal anatomic representation and electromyography enables detection of even small amounts of axon loss, as manifest by fibrillations and positive sharp waves. This enticing approach invites some opposition based on animal[34] and human studies,[35,36] which raise the hypothesis that distal foot muscles may show electrodiagnostic abnormalities due to local muscle trauma attributable to heavy foot use, without peripheral neurologic pathologic condition. However, the nonspecific abnormalities may be reduced with stricter definitions of abnormality, confined to reproducible and sustained positive sharp waves and fibrillations. One study of 70 asymptomatic feet noted positive sharp waves in 8.6%, but found fibrillation potentials much less often, suggesting that not all observed abnormalities carry equal clinical significance.[37] Furthermore, some of these incidentally found abnormalities may, in fact, be clinically relevant, representing true neurologic pathologic condition from conditions not previously diagnosed. Indeed, an electromyographic study of extensor digitorum brevis and abductor hallucis in 20 normal subjects (age range 21–47 years) found abnormalities in 7.[38] However, in 4 cases, alternative explanations of the abnormalities were identified (radiculopathy, sciatic neuropathy, or benign fasciculation syndrome), leaving only 3 cases of isolated abnormality without clinical pathologic explanation; all 3 cases were former athletes. In keeping with these findings, Menkes and Sander[39] report finding prospectively that among patients referred for lower limb studies with positive plantar denervation, the plantar denervation findings were never seen in isolation, and other abnormalities were present when sought. Recently, the fourth dorsal interosseous pedis (DIP) muscle, a different foot intrinsic muscle, has been shown to be frequently abnormal in neuropathy and in S1 radiculopathy, and rarely abnormal in normal controls.[40] Study of the first or fourth DIP muscles is particularly appealing because their dorsal locations on the foot and their distances from bony prominences may render them less susceptible to mechanical or pressure-related trauma from routine activity.

Interpreting Fibular Motor Amplitude on a Functional Basis

Inspection of **Fig. 5**A shows that among older subjects without neuropathy, ankle proprioceptive thresholds become optimally precise when the fibular amplitude exceeds 3.5 to 4.0 mV. Analysis of analogous ankle motor function data also finds that ankle inversion torque generation falls significantly when fibular amplitude is less than 4.0 mV (**Fig. 5**B). Therefore, values <4.0 mV (in the absence of coexisting disease such a proximal compression at the fibular head) can be considered to reflect early peripheral neuromuscular decline, despite exceeding the routinely used "normal" of 2.0 mV.

Taken together, these 3 simple electrodiagnostic techniques may serve to better identify those individuals with suboptimal distal neuromuscular function who carry an increased risk of falls. Clinical relevance is likely enhanced when these measures of distal neuromuscular function are combined with a measure of proximal strength, such as lateral plank time, as described above. In addition to these techniques, serial studies over time may offer valuable insight into the process of neuromuscular decline. Further research should aim to elucidate whether the rate of decline of distal nerve conduction response amplitudes over time holds prognostic value for mobility outcomes and falls risk.

SUCCESSFUL IDENTIFICATION OF EARLY NEUROMUSCULAR DECLINE WILL ENABLE TARGETING FALL RISK INTERVENTIONS

Electrodiagnosticians who successfully identify patients likely to fall will enable clinicians to target advice and interventions to those patients in the highest-risk groups. There are several effective general interventions for reducing falls risk that are applicable to most patients, such as listed in the Centers for Disease Control and Prevention resources.[41] In addition, the electrodiagnostician is well positioned to tailor recommendations to the locus of an individual's most prominent intrinsic impairment, be that the sensory afferent, central neurocognitive, or motor efferent components of response to perturbation. The sensory afferent pathway can be enhanced by optimizing vision or by lightly touching walls or nearby stable objects with the upper limb during walking. To improve executive function and motor planning, one can consider cognitive training ("mindfulness" when walking), attention-enhancing medications, reduction of anticholinergic and other attention-diminishing medication, and evaluation for sleep apnea or other sleep disturbances associated with delayed reaction and/or executive impairments. Finally, to maximize the motor efferent pathways involved in fall prevention, lower limb strengthening (especially the hip region) is targeted, offering ski poles and sport orthoses that increase frontal plane stiffness at the ankle (eg, Active Ankle) for improved lateral control, and weight loss is encouraged when obesity is present. Of note, available data suggest that hip strength can compensate for imprecise foot/ankle proprioceptive function.[15]

SUMMARY

In summary, risk of falls among older adults poses a threat to walking safely—an activity that confers many health and quality-of-life benefits. Understanding the risk factors for falls and development of clinical tools to assess risk will help clinicians appropriately advise patients and target interventions toward those at risk for falls. Distal neuromuscular decline is one of the most important risk domains. Given that this domain represents a continuum of function, with clinical relevance across the continuum, one should aim to develop sound measures of distal neuromuscular function, impairment, and decline. Electrodiagnosticians are poised to develop such measures. The medial plantar nerve conduction study and electromyography of distal foot musculature are 2 techniques that hold promise for increasing the sensitivity for detection of early, but functionally relevant, neuromuscular decline. Furthermore, interpretation of electrodiagnostic data as they pertain to functional outcomes, rather than diagnostic thresholds for disease, adds guiding information. When these strategies are coupled with reliable estimates of strength of key proximal muscles, the electrodiagnostician can provide the patient and referring physician with previously inaccessible, clinically relevant information regarding mobility and fall risk. This information, in turn, will allow the development of specific strategies for the maintenance of optimal function and independence in older populations.

REFERENCES

1. Hakim AA, Petrovitch H, Burchfiel CM, et al. Effects of walking on mortality among nonsmoking retired men. N Engl J Med 1998;338(2):94–9.
2. Manson JE, Hu FB, Rich-Edwards JW, et al. A prospective study of walking as compared with vigorous exercise in the prevention of coronary heart disease in women. N Engl J Med 1999;341(9):650–8.
3. Yaffe K, Barnes D, Nevitt M, et al. A prospective study of physical activity and cognitive decline in elderly women: women who walk. Arch Intern Med 2001; 161(14):1703–8.
4. Rejeski WJ, Ip EH, Bertoni AG, et al. Lifestyle change and mobility in obese adults with type 2 diabetes. N Engl J Med 2012;366(13):1209–17.
5. Boulé NG, Haddad E, Kenny GP, et al. Effects of exercise on glycemic control and body mass in type 2 diabetes mellitus: a meta-analysis of controlled clinical trials. JAMA 2001;286(10):1218–27.
6. Sluik D, Buijsse B, Muckelbauer R, et al. Physical activity and mortality in individuals with diabetes mellitus: a prospective study and meta-analysis. Arch Intern Med 2012;172(17):1285–95.
7. Richardson JK, Hurvitz EA. Peripheral neuropathy: a true risk factor for falls. J Gerontol A Biol Sci Med Sci 1995;50(4):M211–5.
8. Callaghan B, Feldman E. The metabolic syndrome and neuropathy: therapeutic challenges and opportunities. Ann Neurol 2013;74(3):397–403.
9. Cortez M, Singleton JR, Smith AG. Glucose intolerance, metabolic syndrome, and neuropathy. Handb Clin Neurol 2014;126:109–22.
10. Berg WP, Alessio HM, Mills EM, et al. Circumstances and consequences of falls in independent community-dwelling older adults. Age Ageing 1997;6:261–8.
11. Lord SR, Delbaere K, Gandevia SC. Use of a physiologic profile to document motor impairment in ageing and in clinical groups. J Physiol 2016;594:4513–23.
12. Richardson JK. Imbalanced: the confusing circular nature of falls research... and a possible antidote. Am J Phys Med Rehabil 2017;96(1):55–9.
13. Potocanac Z, debruin J, van der Veen S, et al. Fast online corrections of tripping responses. Exp Brain Res 2014;232(11):3579–90.
14. Kearney FC, Harwood RH, Gladman JR, et al. The relationship between executive function and falls and gait abnormalities in older adults: a systematic review. Dement Geriatr Cogn Disord 2013;36(1–2):20–35.
15. Richardson JK, Demott T, Allet L, et al. Hip strength: ankle proprioceptive threshold ratio predicts falls and injury in diabetic neuropathy. Muscle Nerve 2014;50(3):437–42.
16. Ward RE, Caserotti P, Cauley JA, et al. Mobility-related consequences of reduced lower-extremity peripheral nerve function with age: a systematic review. Aging Dis 2016;7(4):466–78.
17. Lange-Maia BS, Cauley JA, Newman AB, et al. Sensorimotor peripheral nerve function and physical activity in older men. J Aging Phys Act 2016;24(4):559–66.
18. Callaghan B, Kerber K, Langa KM, et al. Longitudinal patient-oriented outcomes in neuropathy importance of early detection and falls. Neurology 2015;85(1): 71–9.
19. Andersen H, Gjerstad MD, Jakobsen J. Atrophy of foot muscles. Diabetes Care 2004;27(10):2382–5.
20. Andreassen CS, Jakobsen J, Ringgaard S, et al. Accelerated atrophy of lower leg and foot muscles—a follow-up study of long-term diabetic polyneuropathy using magnetic resonance imaging (MRI). Diabetologia 2009;52(6):1182–91.

21. Kelly LA, Kuitunen S, Racinais S, et al. Recruitment of the plantar intrinsic foot muscles with increasing postural demand. Clin Biomech 2012;27(1):46–51.

22. Ward RE, Boudreau RM, Caserotti P, et al. Sensory and motor peripheral nerve function and incident mobility disability. J Am Geriatr Soc 2014;62(12):2273–9.

23. Richardson JK, Allet L, Kim H, et al. Fibular motor nerve conduction studies and ankle sensorimotor capacities. Muscle Nerve 2013;47(4):497–503.

24. Donaghy A, DeMott T, Allet L, et al. Accuracy of clinical techniques for evaluating lower limb sensorimotor functions associated with increased fall risk. PM R 2016; 8(4):331–9.

25. England JD, Gronseth GS, Franklin G, et al. Distal symmetric polyneuropathy: a definition for clinical research report of the American Academy of Neurology, the American Association of Electrodiagnostic Medicine, and the American Academy of Physical Medicine and Rehabilitation. Neurology 2005;64(2):199–207.

26. Tarulli A. Neuromuscular disease: evidence and analysis in clinical neurology by michael benatar. Semin Neurol 2008;28(02):112 © Thieme Medical Publishers.

27. Rivner MH, Swift TR, Malik K. Influence of age and height on nerve conduction. Muscle Nerve 2001;24(9):1134–41.

28. Løseth S, Nebuchennykh M, Stålberg E, et al. Medial plantar nerve conduction studies in healthy controls and diabetics. Clin Neurophysiol 2007;118(5): 1155–61.

29. Nodera H, Logigian EL, Herrmann DN. Class of nerve fiber involvement in sensory neuropathies: clinical characterization and utility of the plantar nerve action potential. Muscle Nerve 2002;26(2):212–7.

30. Sylantiev C, Schwartz R, Chapman J, et al. Medial plantar nerve testing facilitates identification of polyneuropathy. Muscle Nerve 2008;38(6):1595–8.

31. Herrmann DN, Ferguson ML, Pannoni V, et al. Plantar nerve AP and skin biopsy in sensory neuropathies with normal routine conduction studies. Neurology 2004; 63(5):879–85.

32. Uluc K, Isak B, Borucu D, et al. Medial plantar and dorsal sural nerve conduction studies increase the sensitivity in the detection of neuropathy in diabetic patients. Clin Neurophysiol 2008;119(4):880–5.

33. An JY, Park MS, Kim JS, et al. Comparison of diabetic neuropathy symptom score and medial plantar sensory nerve conduction studies in diabetic patients showing normal routine nerve conduction studies. Intern Med 2008;47(15): 1395–8.

34. Lenman JAR, Ritchie AE. Introduction to clinical electromyography. London: Pitman; 1970. p. 175.

35. Falck BJ, Alaranta H. Fibrillation potentials, positive sharp waves and fasciculation in the intrinsic muscles of the foot in healthy subjects. J Neurol Neurosurg Psychiatry 1983;46(7):681–3.

36. Wiechers D, Guyton JD, Johnson EW. Electromyographic findings in the extensor digitorum brevis in a normal population. Arch Phys Med Rehabil 1976;57(2):84–5.

37. Gatens PF, Saeed MA. Electromyographic findings in the intrinsic muscles of normal feet. Arch Phys Med Rehabil 1982;63(7):317–8.

38. Morgenlander JC, Sanders DB. Spontaneous EMG activity in the extensor digitorum brevis and abductor hallucis muscles in normal subjects. Muscle & nerve 1994;17(11):1346–7.

39. Menkes DL, Sander HW. Plantar muscle fibrillations and positive sharp waves. Muscle & nerve 2000;23(6):989–90.

40. Siddiqi ZA, Nasir A, Ahmed SN. The fourth dorsal interosseus pedis muscle: a useful muscle in routine electromyography. J Clin Neurophysiol 2007;24(6): 444–9.
41. Stevens JA. A CDC compendium of effective fall interventions: what works for community-dwelling older adults. Atlanta (GA): Centers for Disease Control and Prevention (CDC)

Detecting Toxic Myopathies as Medication Side Effect

Elba Gerena-Maldonado, MD*

KEYWORDS

- Toxic myopathy • Rhabdomyolysis • Muscle weakness • Electrodiagnostic studies
- Muscle biopsy

KEY POINTS

- Multiple drugs have been implicated in muscle damage, however, the vast majority of medications are safe if administered in the recommended therapeutic doses.
- Muscle tissue is highly sensitive to drugs and/or toxins due to its high metabolic activity.
- Prompt identification of toxic myopathies is imperative when evaluating a patient with muscle weakness, as these conditions tend to be reversible.
- Comprehensive history and an adequate neuromuscular examination can be complemented with electrodiagnostic studies, MRIs, and muscle biopsies for proper diagnosis and treatment.

INTRODUCTION

Toxic myopathies are described as the acute or subacute manifestation of muscle weakness, myalgia, hyperCKemia, or rhabdomyolysis that can occur in patients without an underlying known muscle disease when they are exposed to certain drugs.[1] Many drug-related myopathies are potentially reversible at early stages[2,3]; however, some of these drugs can have cumulative effects in the muscle and can potentially cause a dose-dependent injury over time to the point of causing irreversible damage.[4] Therefore, early detection of a myopathic process is needed to avoid prolonged exposure to a myotoxic agent. First, the clinician must always elicit a thorough history and perform a comprehensive neuromuscular examination. Second, when considering an electrodiagnostic study evaluation in the setting of a suspected myopathy, the clinician should consider this tool as simply an extension of the clinical examination of the patient. Although helpful in demonstrating the presence of a myopathic process, these studies tend to be more useful by excluding other potential causes for muscle

Disclosure Statement: Nothing to disclose.
Department of Physical Medicine and Rehabilitation, Providence St. Joseph Health, Providence Medical Group, 500 West Broadway, 3rd Floor, Missoula, MT 59802, USA
* Corresponding author. Physical Medicine and Rehabilitation Clinic, 500 West Broadway, 3rd Floor, Missoula, MT 59802.
E-mail address: Elba.GerenaMaldonado@providence.org

Phys Med Rehabil Clin N Am 29 (2018) 659–667
https://doi.org/10.1016/j.pmr.2018.06.002
1047-9651/18/© 2018 Elsevier Inc. All rights reserved.

weakness, such as polyneuropathy, motor neuron disease, or neuromuscular junction disorders.[5]

ELECTRODIAGNOSTIC EVALUATION FOR SUSPECTED MYOPATHY

The following are the recommended guidelines for the nerve conduction studies and electromyography (EMG) when evaluating a patient with a suspected myopathy[6]:

- At least 1 sensory nerve in 1 upper and 1 lower limb. If studies are abnormal, more extensive evaluation is required.
- At least 1 motor nerve in 1 upper and 1 lower limb.
- Needle EMG of proximal and distal muscles in 1 upper and 1 lower limb and thoracic paraspinals. If motor units appear myopathic, this may be studied further by quantitative evaluation of motor unit action potentials.
- Repetitive nerve stimulation and single-fiber EMG can be considered if a neuromuscular junction disorder is suspected.
- If a muscle biopsy is being considered, avoid performing an EMG in the muscle on which the biopsy is to be performed.

IMAGING AND BIOPSY FOR SUSPECTED MYOPATHY

Muscle biopsies and MRI are additional diagnostic tools, which if used appropriately, can be valuable in identifying and further characterizing the potential structural and neurophysiological abnormalities in skeletal muscle.

In particular, MRI of skeletal muscle has been found helpful in localizing the specific muscles affected in patients presenting with acute/subacute muscle weakness.[7] Key patterns have been identified in the MRI evaluation of myopathy, including abnormal anatomy with normal signal intensity, edema or inflammation, and muscle atrophy. Muscle edema, although the most common pattern found, is nonspecific and carries a broad differential diagnosis.[8] However, for example, autoimmune, paraneoplastic, and drug-induced myositis tend to present with symmetric areas of edema, whereas infection, radiation-induced injury, and myonecrosis are focal asymmetric processes. MRI features, when correlated with clinical and laboratory findings, as well as findings from other methods such as EMG, may facilitate correct diagnosis.[8,9]

Another imaging tool that is noninvasive, inexpensive, and useful in evaluating muscle disease is neuromuscular ultrasound. Ultrasound allows for assessment of muscle thickness, abnormal movements (eg, fasciculations), and infiltration of fat or fibrotic tissue. It can also evaluate inflammation in muscle and differentiate between a neurogenic inflammatory pattern versus myopathic pattern as the cause of muscle weakness.[10]

Although the presumptive diagnosis of skeletal muscle disease may be made on the basis of clinical-radiological correlation with supportive evidence from electrodiagnostic studies, in many cases, muscle biopsy is often required to confirm the diagnosis. Muscle biopsies are associated with highly positive diagnostic outcome in the presence of hyperCKemia, proximal weakness, and myopathic EMG findings. However, in the absence of myopathic EMG and/or proximal weakness, the chance of finding specific myopathy with a muscle biopsy is generally low, regardless of the creatine kinase (CK) level.[11]

CLINICAL SYNDROMES AND SUBTYPES OF TOXIC MYOPATHIES

Myopathies are classified as hereditary or acquired and are further subcategorized depending on their clinical and pathologic findings (**Table 1**). It is important to highlight

Table 1	
Classification of most common myopathies	
Hereditary Myopathies	**Acquired Myopathies**
Muscular dystrophies	Inflammatory myopathies
Congenital myopathies	Toxic myopathies
Distal myopathies	Endocrine myopathies
Mitochondrial myopathies	Myopathies secondary to systemic diseases
Metabolic myopathies	
Channelopathies	

that toxic myopathies represent a fraction of all the potential myopathic processes known to date in the pediatric and adult population.[12] One of the first steps in identifying the cause of any neurologic syndrome is to identify exposure to a potentially reversible toxic agent that could incite injury. The most common toxic agents associated with myopathy include statins and other lipid-lowering medications, corticosteroids, colchicine, amiodarone, hydroxychloroquine, and chloroquine. The following sections are divided in the most common clinical syndromes associated with toxic myopathies and the agents associated with these conditions.

Rhabdomyolysis Syndrome

The criteria for diagnosing rhabdomyolysis can vary depending on the reference source. Nevertheless, it is generally considered an acute syndrome due to extensive injury of the skeletal muscle in which there is necrosis or permeabilization of sarcolemma with release of muscle proteins into circulation (usually serum CK: >10,000). This is usually associated with proximal muscle weakness, myalgia, swelling, and in more severe cases, with myoglobinuria, cardiomyopathy, encephalopathy, and death. Muscle tissue is sensitive to drugs and toxins because of its high metabolic activity and the potential for drugs to disrupt these metabolic pathways. The following are some of the more common agents associated with rhabdomyolysis syndrome.

Ethanol

Alcoholic myopathy may manifest as an acute or chronic condition. Chronic alcohol-related myopathy is the most common presentation in the clinical setting and it is estimated to be 10 times more common than the most common inherited myopathies.[13] Clinically, acute alcoholic myopathy is characterized by a rhabdomyolysis syndrome with an acute presentation of weakness, pain, and swelling of affected muscles (trunk muscles > appendicular muscles). It often occurs after a single episode of alcohol binge drinking and resolves within 1 to 2 weeks of abstinence from alcohol.[14] EMG findings with the acute myopathy presentation tend to include fibrillation potentials and positive sharp waves with brief small abundant polyphasic motor unit action potentials on recruitment.[15]

Chronic heavy alcohol consumption can lead to protein calorie malnutrition, which frequently is related to the severity of alcoholic liver disease. Chronic alcoholic myopathy is characterized by decreased protein synthesis of both myofibrillar and sarcoplasmic proteins.[16] Nowadays, the advances made in the fields of cell biology and biochemistry have identified the molecular pathways contributing to alcohol-induced muscle wasting. These include the following: reductions in mammalian target of rapamycin–mediated protein synthesis and excessive protein degradation by activation of the Ubiquitin Proteasome Pathway and autophagic-lysosomal system. It is thought that in the setting of acute inflammation, oxidative stress, and mitochondrial dysfunction, the exacerbation of these pathways is associated with accelerated muscle wasting.[4] Clinical presentation of these patients includes muscle wasting, proximal muscle weakness, with associated liver cirrhosis, potential cardiomyopathy, and nutritional deficiencies. Electrodiagnostic findings in the chronic form of alcoholic myopathy usually demonstrate an axonal sensorimotor polyneuropathy and normal needle EMG findings.[15] Muscle biopsies tend to show type II fiber atrophy, muscle fiber necrosis, and regeneration intersegmental manner, separation of myelofibrosis, tubular aggregates, and moth-eaten muscle fibers.

Opiates

Rhabdomyolysis syndrome occurs at a relatively high rate in acute poisonings. Depending on the agent's toxicity, severe rhabdomyolysis and its complications may significantly influence the patient's clinical course and prognosis. In one case series, a retrospective review of a 1-year period evaluated 656 cases of rhabdomyolysis caused by acute poisoning at the Clinic for Emergency and Clinical Toxicology of the Military Medical Academy, in Belgrade, Serbia. The study found that the highest percentage (41%) of rhabdomyolysis cases caused by poisoning was secondary to opiates.[17] Another large series evaluated 475 patients with rhabdomyolysis admitted to the medicine ward in Baltimore, MD, and their findings were that the most common cause of rhabdomyolysis was secondary to illicit drugs, alcohol, and prescribed drugs, which accounted for 46% of those admissions.[18] The increased risk of rhabdomyolysis with each of these substances has been attributed to direct toxic effect of the drug or contaminants, increased sympathomimetic stimulation, and/or nutritional deficiency in the setting of addiction. Given its prevalence, obtaining a history of substance use is a critical part of a rhabdomyolysis evaluation.[19] In these cases, the clinical presentation of the patient can range from muscle abscess, induration, and muscle contracture from fibrosis, and muscle ischemia. The CKs can range from normal to elevated, depending on the clinical presentation (chronic muscle fibrosis vs rhabdomyolysis). EMG findings will demonstrate fibrillation potentials, positive sharp waves, and brief small abundant polyphasic motor unit action potentials in necrotic muscle.[15]

Cholesterol-lowering agents

The frequency of myopathy with cholesterol-lowering agents has been found to be approximately 1 to 6 in 10,000.[20,21] Risk factors include female gender, patients who are 70 years or older, and associated renal, liver disease, or diabetes. Usual onset of symptoms is after 2 to 3 months of starting lipid-lowering drug. Among the most common clinical presentations are complaints of myalgias that are present at rest and worsen with exercise, muscle weakness, and myoglobinuria. Usually the serum CK levels are elevated and the muscle biopsy findings will reveal scattered necrotic muscle fibers. Two main cholesterol-lowering agents have been identified as potentially causing toxic myopathies, fibrates, and statins.

Fibrates or fibric acid derivatives, such as clofibrate, fenofibrate, and gemfibrozil have been found to have a relative risk of 42.4 times more likely of precipitating a toxic myopathy in patients who take this class of medications than nonusers.[22] The primary metabolism of this medication class is renal, and patients who have a concomitant renal failure or use other medications, such as furosemide or statins, are at a higher risk of developing a toxic myopathy and rhabdomyolysis.[23,24] Some of the fibrates have been associated with a higher risk of myopathy; fenofibrate being the least likely to cause rhabdomyolysis.

Statins, or 3-hydroxy-3-methylglutaryl-coenzyme A (HMG-CoA) reductase inhibitors, have been proven to reduce the risk of cardiovascular disease in patients with hyperlipidemia. One of the main reasons for patients to be noncompliant with this class of medications is because of the side effects of myalgias (most common clinical syndrome associated with statins). All of the statins available in the market have been associated with some form of myopathic disorder. The relative toxicity of these medications correlates with their half-life; the longer the half-life, the higher the relative myotoxicity. The spectrum of myopathic disorders associated with statins includes asymptomatic hyperCKemia, myalgia, toxic necrotizing myopathy, immune-mediated necrotizing myopathy, and rhabdomyolysis. Routine motor and sensory nerve conduction studies should be normal. Needle EMG can demonstrate fibrillation potentials, positive sharp waves, and early recruitment of short-duration motor unit action potentials on those patients with significant muscle weakness. Possible direct mechanisms underlying myopathy secondary to statin include altered skeletal muscle cell membrane permeability; reduced levels of ubiquinone, and reduction in the synthesis of coenzyme Q10.

One of the rare ($\sim$2 of every 100,000 patients treated with statins) but serious side effects of statin use is statin-associated autoimmune myopathy. These patients present with symmetric proximal muscle weakness, which usually persists or worsens even if statin therapy is discontinued. The serum CK levels tend to exceed 2000 IU per liter and the EMG shows small-amplitude motor unit potentials with increased spontaneous activity characteristic of an active (irritable) myopathic process. MRI tends to demonstrate edema on the proximal muscles that are affected. It is the muscle biopsy that provides the visible muscle-cell necrosis and regeneration. The muscle biopsy also will demonstrate autoantibodies against HMG-CoA reductase. Anti-HMG-CoA reductase autoantibodies have not been detected in statin-treated patients who do not have muscle disease or in whom dose in home self-limited statin–related myopathy develop. Therefore, in patients who have myopathy after statin any exposure, a positive test for anti-HMG-CoA reductase autoantibodies strongly supports the diagnosis of an autoimmune disease.[25,26] Current theory suggests that statin-induced overexpression of HMG-CoA reductase in genetically susceptible patients may cause autoimmunity against HMG-CoA reductase. Confirmation of the diagnosis with a test for anti–HMG-CoA reductase autoantibody should lead to the discontinuation of treatment with statins and the initiation of immunosuppressive therapy. When this disorder is recognized and treated, patients with statin-associated autoimmune myopathy usually have a good outcomes.[27]

The management of intolerance to lipid-lowering medications is challenging in patients who require treatment for dyslipidemia. For patients who require a medication for dyslipidemia, use of a different statin or different class of lipid-lowering medication can be considered, but the risk of recurrence of myopathic symptoms or elevated serum CK may be high (15% or higher).[28]

Myosin Deficiency (Thick-Filament Loss) Myopathies

This phenomenon is also known as rapidly evolving myopathy with myosin-deficient fibers, critical-illness myopathy, or acute quadriplegia. It can be associated to the exposure of high doses of corticosteroids or neuromuscular junction blocking agents, usually in the intensive care unit setting. The typical clinical presentation of these patients is a progressive proximal > distal muscle weakness over days to weeks, sometimes with persistent weakness after respiratory support or exposure to neuromuscular junction blocking agents. Slow improvement in muscle weakness can be observed when steroids are tapered. This diagnosis does carry a high mortality (up to 50%) rate, usually from associated disorders. Laboratory findings can include normal or elevated serum CK levels and electrodiagnostic studies demonstrate reduced amplitude in the compound motor action potential with normal conduction velocity and distal latencies; sensory potentials tend to be normal, and the EMG findings can be normal or demonstrate positive sharp waves and fibrillation potentials early in the course with short-duration, small-amplitude, polyphasic motor unit action potentials that recruited early are evident.[15] The muscle biopsy will demonstrate myosin loss in muscle fibers on ATPase stain (ATPase, pH 9.4 and 4.3), atrophic muscle fibers, degeneration and regeneration of muscle fibers, and reduced NOS1 (nNOS) staining in the sarcolemma.

When considering glucocorticoid-induced myopathy, we also must be cognizant of the chronic form of its presentation. In chronic steroid myopathy, muscle weakness develops insidiously, progresses slowly, and is usually painless or mildly painful.[29] Glucocorticoid-induced muscle atrophy affects fast-twitch (type II) glycolytic muscle fibers.[30] Clinically, the patient will present with a proximal muscle weakness, most commonly involving the hip girdle muscles. Electrodiagnostic studies usually demonstrate normal motor and sensory nerve conduction studies. The needle EMG typically is normal unless the myopathy is severe. It is important to point out that abnormal spontaneous activity is not seen. Therefore, if the EMG study presents with abundant abnormal spontaneous activity, it may strongly suggest that an inflammatory myopathy is the underlying cause of the muscle weakness and not the steroid medication. Please refer to **Box 1** for a list of toxic myopathies with increased spontaneous activity features on EMG.

It is thought that the catabolic effect of glucocorticoids on muscle proteolysis results from the activation of the major cellular proteolytic systems, including the ubiquitin-proteasome system, the lysosomal system, and the calcium-dependent system.[31] The treatment for this type of myopathy is to reduce the steroid dose, alternate day treatment regimen, and/or switching to a nonfluorinated agent (prednisone or methylprednisolone). A combination of changes between the medical treatment and working with physical therapy alongside will help to avoid muscle wasting in this patient population.[32]

Mitochondrial Myopathies

Certain antiviral medications can cause toxicity to myocytes via decreased mitochondrial DNA expression and subsequent mitochondrial toxicity. This includes selected antiretroviral medications used for treatment of human immunodeficiency virus (HIV), such as zidovudine (AZT), a nucleoside reverse transcriptase inhibitor. AZT myopathy must usually be distinguished from HIV-associated myopathy. The exact incidence is varied between studies but is approximately 5% to 10% in patients taking

---

Box 1
Toxic myopathies with spontaneous activity on electromyography

Colchicine

Zidovudine (AZT)

Alcohol

Chloroquine

Hydroxychloroquine

Cholesterol-lowering agents

Critical-illness myopathy

AZT. This myopathy typically presents with proximal weakness and myalgias[33] after treatment for usually 1 year. Laboratory findings include elevated serum CK values, which vary from 2 to 10 times normal. Electrophysiological findings include normal motor and sensory nerve conductions studies (unless there is a concomitant peripheral neuropathy from the disease). Needle examination has been reported to demonstrate increased insertional activity with positive sharp waves and fibrillation potentials, and occasional complex repetitive discharges. On recruitment, the pattern observed is of early recruitment of short-duration small-amplitude polyphasic motor unit action potentials, usually in proximal muscles.[15] The muscle biopsy findings usually include fiber size variation, some inflammation and necrosis, succinate dehydrogenase–positive and cytochrome oxidase–negative muscle fibers with cytoplasmic bodies. The patient's muscle weakness usually improves after discontinuation of drug, within 3 to 4 months.

Vacuolar Myopathies

Chloroquine, hydroxychloroquine, and amiodarone are also known as amphiphilic drugs, which may cause a lysosomal storage disorder and increased autophagosome formation. In general, patients who suffer from a vacuolar myopathy secondary to these medications will present with a proximal greater than distal myopathy that may be associated with a cardiomyopathy or a neuropathy. The serum CK levels can be mildly elevated. Electrodiagnostic findings can demonstrate mild slowing of both motor and sensory nerve conduction study velocities with mild reduction in amplitudes, and slightly prolonged F-waves if there is a superimposed neuropathy. On needle EMG, positive sharp waves and fibrillation potentials are usually seen on proximal limb muscles. Small-amplitude, short-duration, polyphasic voluntary motor unit action potentials have been seen on recruitment, and in the case of chloroquine, there have been reported myotonic potentials despite the lack of clinical myotonia.[15,34] The muscle biopsy will demonstrate acid-phosphatase vacuoles, normal periodic acid-Schiff staining for glycogen, and electromicroscopy demonstrating curvilinear and myeloid bodies. Slow recovery is expected once the offending medication is discontinued.[35]

SUMMARY

Toxic exposures are important etiologies to consider in all patients with myopathy because these conditions are often reversible with prompt treatment or removal of the offending agent. Medication combinations can also lead to myotoxicity and myopathy. It is important to distinguish between muscle disease secondary to illness (ie, autoimmune, inflammatory, or infectious cause) and muscle weakness secondary to the toxicity from medications. It is for this reason that it is imperative that the clinician is able to elicit a thorough history and physical examination on these patients. Electrodiagnostic studies play an important role in excluding competing diagnoses, confirming a suspected clinical diagnosis of myopathy, and occasionally providing clues for categories of myopathy based on the presence or absence of abnormal spontaneous activity. An understanding of the utility and limitation of the diagnostic tests available will help narrow the differential diagnosis and potentially confirm a specific etiology of muscle disease.

REFERENCES

1. Dalakas MC. Toxic and drug-induced myopathies. J Neurol Neurosurg Psychiatry 2009;80(8):832–8.

2. Echaniz-Laguna A, Mohr M, Tranchant C. Neuromuscular symptoms and elevated creatine kinase after statin withdrawal. N Engl J Med 2010;362(6):564–5.

3. Hansen KE, Hildebrand JP, Ferguson EE, et al. Outcomes in 45 patients with statin-associated myopathy. Arch Intern Med 2005;165(22):2671–6.

4. Simon L, Jolley SE, Molina PE. Alcoholic myopathy: pathophysiologic mechanisms and clinical implications. Alcohol Res 2017;38(2):207–17.

5. Chahin N, Sorenson EJ. Serum creatine kinase levels in spinobulbar muscular atrophy and amyotrophic lateral sclerosis. Muscle Nerve 2009;40(1):126–9.

6. Srinivasan J, Amato AA. Myopathies. Phys Med Rehabil Clin N Am 2003;14(2):403–34, x.

7. Sookhoo S, Mackinnon I, Bushby K, et al. MRI for the demonstration of subclinical muscle involvement in muscular dystrophy. Clin Radiol 2007;62(2):160–5.

8. Smitaman E, Flores DV, Mejía Gómez C, et al. MR imaging of atraumatic muscle disorders. Radiographics 2018;38(2):500–22.

9. Theodorou DJ, Theodorou SJ, Kakitsubata Y. Skeletal muscle disease: patterns of MRI appearances. Br J Radiol 2012;85(1020):e1298–308.

10. Pillen S, Arts IM, Zwarts MJ. Muscle ultrasound in neuromuscular disorders. Muscle Nerve 2008;37(6):679–93.

11. Shaibani A, Jabari D, Jabbour M, et al. Diagnostic outcome of muscle biopsy. Muscle Nerve 2015;51(5):662–8.

12. Echaniz-Laguna A, Mohr M, Lannes B, et al. Myopathies in the elderly: a hospital-based study. Neuromuscul Disord 2010;20(7):443–7.

13. Preedy VR, Ohlendieck K, Adachi J, et al. The importance of alcohol-induced muscle disease. J Muscle Res Cell Motil 2003;24(1):55–63.

14. Riggs JE. Alcohol-associated rhabdomyolysis: ethanol induction of cytochrome P450 may potentiate myotoxicity. Clin Neuropharmacol 1998;21(6):363–4.

15. Dumitru D. Electrodiagnostic medicine. 2002.

16. Steiner JL, Lang CH. Dysregulation of skeletal muscle protein metabolism by alcohol. Am J Physiol Endocrinol Metab 2015;308(9):E699–712.

17. Jankovic SR, Stosić JJ, Vucinić S, et al. Causes of rhabdomyolysis in acute poisonings. Vojnosanit Pregl 2013;70(11):1039–45.

18. Melli G, Chaudhry V, Cornblath DR. Rhabdomyolysis: an evaluation of 475 hospitalized patients. Medicine (Baltimore) 2005;84(6):377–85.

19. Nance JR, Mammen AL. Diagnostic evaluation of rhabdomyolysis. Muscle Nerve 2015;51(6):793–810.

20. Law M, Rudnicka AR. Statin safety: a systematic review. Am J Cardiol 2006;97(8A):52C–60C.

21. Ganga HV, Slim HB, Thompson PD. A systematic review of statin-induced muscle problems in clinical trials. Am Heart J 2014;168(1):6–15.

22. Gaist D, Rodríguez LA, Huerta C, et al. Lipid-lowering drugs and risk of myopathy: a population-based follow-up study. Epidemiology 2001;12(5):565–9.

23. Soyoral YU, Canbaz ET, Erdur MF, et al. Fenofibrate-induced rhabdomyolysis in a patient with stage 4 chronic renal failure due to diabetes mellitus. J Pak Med Assoc 2012;62(8):849–51.

24. Forcadell-Peris MJ, de Diego-Cabanes C. Rhabdomyolysis secondary to simvastatin and phenofibrate. Semergen 2014;40(4):e91–4 [in Spanish].

25. Mammen AL, Chung T, Christopher-Stine L, et al. Autoantibodies against 3-hydroxy-3-methylglutaryl-coenzyme A reductase in patients with statin-associated autoimmune myopathy. Arthritis Rheum 2011;63(3):713–21.

26. Mammen AL, Pak K, Williams EK, et al. Rarity of anti-3-hydroxy-3-methylglutaryl-coenzyme A reductase antibodies in statin users, including those with self-limited musculoskeletal side effects. Arthritis Care Res (Hoboken) 2012;64(2):269–72.
27. Mammen AL. Statin-associated autoimmune myopathy. N Engl J Med 2016; 374(7):664–9.
28. Fung EC, Crook MA. Statin myopathy: a lipid clinic experience on the tolerability of statin rechallenge. Cardiovasc Ther 2012;30(5):e212–8.
29. Pereira RM, Freire de Carvalho J. Glucocorticoid-induced myopathy. Joint Bone Spine 2011;78(1):41–4.
30. Schakman O, Gilson H, Thissen JP. Mechanisms of glucocorticoid-induced myopathy. J Endocrinol 2008;197(1):1–10.
31. Hasselgren PO. Glucocorticoids and muscle catabolism. Curr Opin Clin Nutr Metab Care 1999;2(3):201–5.
32. Gupta A, Gupta Y. Glucocorticoid-induced myopathy: pathophysiology, diagnosis, and treatment. Indian J Endocrinol Metab 2013;17(5):913–6.
33. Dalakas MC, Pezeshkpour GH. Neuromuscular diseases associated with human immunodeficiency virus infection. Ann Neurol 1988;23(Suppl):S38–48.
34. Estes ML, Ewing-Wilson D, Chou SM, et al. Chloroquine neuromyotoxicity. Clinical and pathologic perspective. Am J Med 1987;82(3):447–55.
35. Flanagan EP, Harper CM, St Louis EK, et al. Amiodarone-associated neuromyopathy: a report of four cases. Eur J Neurol 2012;19(5):e50–1.

Electrodiagnostic Testing for the Diagnosis and Management of Amyotrophic Lateral Sclerosis

Ileana M. Howard, MD[a],*, Nassim Rad, MD[b]

KEYWORDS

- Amyotrophic lateral sclerosis • Electrodiagnosis • Motor neuron disease
- Biomarkers • X-linked bulbospinal atrophy

KEY POINTS

- Careful history and physical examinations should guide a thorough diagnostic evaluation, with laboratory and electrodiagnostic studies to exclude the possibility of treatable mimic diseases.
- The Awaji modifications to the El Escorial diagnostic criteria have increased the sensitivity for diagnosis of amyotrophic lateral sclerosis by making electromyography findings of equal importance to clinical examination findings.
- Evidence of subclinical disease by electromyography in clinically normal muscles can foreshadow progression of weakness and relate to poorer prognosis.
- Diaphragmatic denervation on needle electromyography may suggest impaired neuromuscular respiratory function and should trigger evaluation to maximize respiratory management.
- Several electrodiagnostic measures have been proposed as biomarkers to monitor progression and may be useful measures for research or clinical use to assess response to disease-modifying medications.

INTRODUCTION

Amyotrophic lateral sclerosis (ALS) is the most common adult-onset motor neuron disease with an estimated prevalence of approximately 3.9 per 100,000 persons in the United States.[1] Despite the classic presentation of mixed upper and lower motor neuron signs and symptoms, a great deal of phenotypic heterogeneity exists in ALS, which adds to the challenge in establishing a diagnosis.[2–6] Electrodiagnostic testing provides key insight into subclinical aspects of disease in ALS. For this reason,

Disclosure: None.
[a] Rehabilitation Care Medicine, VA Puget Sound Healthcare System, S-117 RCS, 1660 South Columbian Way, Seattle, WA 98108, USA; [b] Department of Rehabilitation Medicine, University of Washington, 325 Ninth Avenue, Box 359612, Seattle, WA 98104, USA
* Corresponding author.
E-mail address: ileana.howard@va.gov

Phys Med Rehabil Clin N Am 29 (2018) 669–680
https://doi.org/10.1016/j.pmr.2018.06.003
1047-9651/18/Published by Elsevier Inc.

it serves an important role in establishing the diagnosis and excluding other competing diagnoses. Although some investigators may limit consideration of electrodiagnostic testing in ALS only to the role of confirming a clinical diagnosis, to stop there may prematurely constrain the full usefulness of this tool. Electrodiagnostic testing may provide useful information to guide management or track disease progression. Mapping the extent of subclinical disease may help to guide the clinician to appropriate supportive interventions. Finally, there is considerable interest in establishing biomarkers to monitor progression of disease over time. Electrodiagnostic biomarkers have the benefit of being more sensitive to change than traditionally used outcome measures and do not require specialized equipment.

This article details the usefulness of electrodiagnostic testing across the disease spectrum in ALS, including to establish a diagnosis, identify common ALS mimic disorders, monitor progression for ongoing management, and predict prognosis. Before delving into specific electrodiagnostic studies for motor neuron disease, a brief review of clinical presentations and differential diagnoses is presented. Emerging applications of electrodiagnostic studies to guide management and assess response to treatment interventions are then presented. We conclude with considerations for clinical practice.

CLINICAL PRESENTATION OF AMYOTROPHIC LATERAL SCLEROSIS

The heterogeneity of clinical presentation in ALS often leads to long delays between the onset of symptoms and a diagnosis, which in turn limits access to disease-modifying medications and investigational therapeutics, as well as supportive interventions that may prolong life expectancy, improve quality of life, or maintain function. Major advances in disease awareness have done little to decrease the diagnostic lag time. A delay of 1 year between symptom onset and diagnosis is still common; 1 study found no evidence of improvement in this metric in Great Britain over a 20-year period despite efforts to fast track evaluations for suspected motor neuron disease.[7]

Initial symptoms of weakness may present in the limbs (~60%), bulbar muscles (~30%), or, more rarely, in the respiratory muscles (~3%). Weakness is generally asymmetric and progresses regionally to adjacent myotomes and body regions; however, some variants of ALS demonstrate prolonged periods of disease isolated to a single body region, for example, in brachial amyotrophy (Hiramaya disease). Bulbar weakness may present as dysphagia or dysarthria. Respiratory weakness is common as the disease progresses; initial symptoms may be subtle and involve orthopnea or sleep-disordered breathing. Although cognition and behavior was once thought to be spared from the disease process in ALS, frontotemporal dementia is now recognized as part of the disease spectrum[8]; symptoms may either precede muscle weakness or manifest with disease progression. Other signs and symptoms frequently associated with ALS are weight loss, fatigue, and musculoskeletal complaints. Although not thought to be a common presenting feature of ALS, pain is reported in about one-half of all patients as a consequence of muscle imbalance and progressive loss of muscle mass and mobility.[9] Common pain complaints include shoulder pain, back and neck pain, and pain related to medical procedures (gastrostomy, tracheostomy tube placement). Neuropathic pain, however, is an uncommonly reported symptom in persons with ALS.

The evaluation of a patient suspected of having ALS begins with a detailed history and physical examination. Cranial nerve function, sensory examination, and cerebellar examinations should be normal. Bladder and bowel function are generally intact. Weakness, atrophy, hypotonia, hyporeflexia, and fasciculations are signs of lower motor neuron pathology. Neck extensor weakness is a manifestation of muscle weakness often seen in ALS, although it is not pathognomonic. Upper motor neuron signs on examination may include spasticity and hyperreflexia, indicated by abnormal spread of reflexes and clonus or by the presence of brisk reflexes in regions of muscle atrophy. Pathologic reflexes, such as the Babinski sign, Hoffmann sign, and a hyperactive jaw jerk are also highly suggestive of upper motor neuron dysfunction.

DIFFERENTIAL DIAGNOSIS

Several disorders may present with overlapping symptoms to ALS and should be considered and excluded during the diagnostic evaluation. These disorders include those of the central and peripheral nervous systems and other neuromuscular disorders. An appropriate differential diagnosis is crafted based on individual clinical presentation, with special consideration for common ALS mimic disorders.

Central nervous system disorders, such as brain or spinal cord pathology, must be considered in the presence of mixed upper and motor lower neuron signs. Other anterior horn cell/motor neuron diseases that may be considered include adult-onset spinal muscular atrophy, X-linked spinobulbar muscular atrophy (Kennedy's disease), primary lateral sclerosis, and primary muscular atrophy. Although primary lateral sclerosis and primary muscular atrophy were previously thought to be easily distinguishable from classic ALS, current evidence suggest that these disorders exist along a spectrum with the classic mixed upper motor neuron/lower motor neuron presentation of ALS. Among peripheral nerve disorders, multifocal motor neuropathy (MMN) with conduction block and other pure motor neuropathies, such as acute motor axonal neuropathy, should be considered owing to similarities in presentation with ALS. A clinical presentation of both motor and sensory impairments should expand the differential diagnosis to include sensorimotor peripheral neuropathies. Neuromuscular junction disorders—in particular Lambert-Eaton myasthenic syndrome and myasthenia gravis—should be considered, particularly if a history of fatiguable weakness is obtained. Finally, myopathies should also be strongly considered in the setting of ALS, particularly if reflexes are intact or only slightly diminished. Inclusion body myositis is a common acquired myopathy often seen in a similar age demographic to individuals with ALS.

DIAGNOSTIC TESTING FOR AMYOTROPHIC LATERAL SCLEROSIS

In the absence of reliable biomarkers, ALS remains a clinical diagnosis supported by electrodiagnostic findings. Despite the increased availability of genetic testing for genes related to ALS, there is no diagnostic test that can confirm the diagnosis. The diagnosis of ALS and other forms of adult motor neuron disease, therefore, is primarily a process of exclusion. Patients with early or limited disease may prove challenging to diagnose, another contributing factor to diagnostic delays.[10]

Initial electrodiagnostic testing can be helpful to confirm a clinically suspected diagnosis of motor neuron disease, to exclude competing and possibly treatable diagnoses (such as MMN with conduction blocks), and to define the extent of the disease process. Motor nerve conduction studies may be normal or may reveal decreased amplitudes with relatively preserved latencies and conduction velocities. With significant loss of amplitude, a 25% decrease in conduction velocity is allowable, given the possible loss of the fastest conducting nerve fibers. Sensory nerve conduction studies are generally normal in ALS. Repetitive stimulation may show an abnormal decrement in ALS; it has been proposed that this feature may be helpful in distinguishing ALS from cervical spondylotic myelopathy[11] and Hiramaya disease.[12] Needle electrode examination provides the most information for detailing the extent of the disease and providing electrodiagnostic data in support of the diagnosis. Needle electromyography (EMG) assesses lower motor neuron involvement, including emerging subclinical disease. Abnormal spontaneous activity, including fibrillation potentials, positive sharp waves, and fasciculations, may be observed. Motor unit action potentials may exhibit polyphasia, increased amplitude and duration, and reduced recruitment. Careful muscle selection can increase the sensitivity of the electrodiagnostic study to detect ALS. In particular, distal limb muscles (first dorsal interosseous, abductor digiti minimi, and abductor pollicis brevis in the upper extremity; tibialis anterior and posterior, medial gastrocnemius, and flexor digitorum longus in the lower extremity) have the greatest likelihood of abnormalities in persons with ALS, regardless of the site of onset of symptoms; an algorithm based on these findings has been proposed in an effort to prioritize the muscles with highest sensitivity within a segment and limit the number of muscles necessary to establish a diagnosis.[13]

Electrodiagnostic criteria to support the clinical suspicion of ALS have evolved over time. The most well-known criteria are the El Escorial Criteria—Revised (**Table 1**). These criteria were established and then updated by The World Federation of Neurology in an effort to define consensus criteria for enrollment into clinical trials and research studies related to ALS.[14] The criteria outlined threshold requirements to establish a diagnosis of definite, probable, probable laboratory—supported, or possible ALS (the category of suspected ALS included in the original El Escorial Criteria was deleted from the revised version). According to the revised El Escorial Criteria, the diagnosis of ALS requires the presence of lower motor neuron degeneration (by clinical, electrophysiologic, or neuropathologic examination), evidence of upper motor neuron degeneration by clinical examination, and progressive spread of symptoms or signs within a region or to other regions.[14] At the same time, the criteria require the absence of electrophysiologic, radiologic, or pathologic evidence of disease processes that might mimic the observed signs of lower motor neuron and/or upper motor neuron degeneration.[14] Electrodiagnostic studies can be used to provide laboratory evidence of lower motor neuron dysfunction: to meet criteria, one must obtain evidence of both active denervation (defined as fibrillations and positive sharp waves) and chronic reinnervation (defined as long duration, large amplitude motor units with reduced recruitment) in 2 of 4 separate body regions (bulbar, cervical, thoracic, and lumbosacral).[14] Of note, these changes must be seen in at least

Table 1 El Escorial criteria—revised	
Diagnostic Category	**Requirements**
Clinically definite ALS	UMN + LMN signs on clinical examination in 3 body regions
Clinically probable ALS	UMN + LMN signs on clinical examination in 2 body regions, with some UMN signs rostral to the LMN signs
Clinically probable ALS – laboratory supported	UMN + LMN signs on clinical examination in 1 body region, OR UMN signs alone in 1 region, AND LMN signs defined by EMG criteria are present in at least 2 regions
Possible ALS	UMN + LMN signs in 1 body region, OR UMN signs in 2 or more body regions, OR LMN signs rostral to UMN signs, AND the diagnosis of clinically probable ALS – laboratory supported cannot be proven

Abbreviations: ALS, amyotrophic lateral sclerosis; body regions, bulbar, cervical, thoracic, lumbosacral; LMN, lower motor neuron; UMN, upper motor neuron.

Data from Brooks BR, Miller RG, Swash M, et al. El Escorial revisited: revised criteria for the diagnosis of amyotrophic lateral sclerosis. Amyotroph Lateral Scler Other Motor Neuron Disord 2000;1(5):293–9.

2 muscles innervated by different roots and peripheral nerves when the cervical and lumbosacral regions are examined. In the bulbar region, changes in 1 muscle would suffice. In the thoracic region, changes either in the paraspinal muscles at or below the T6 level or in the abdominal muscles are acceptable. Again, the revised El Escorial Criteria were established mostly for research purposes and trial enrollment and are strict at a cost to the sensitivity of this measure; 1 population-based study found 10% of persons with ALS died without ever meeting threshold criteria for diagnosis.[15]

The Awaji Electrodiagnostic Criteria for diagnosis of ALS were introduced in 2008 to increase testing sensitivity as compared with the revised El Escorial Criteria (**Table 2**). These criteria confer more weight to electrodiagnostic findings by allowing fasciculation potentials in the setting of polyphasic motor unit action potentials to be considered equivalent to fibrillations as signs of acute denervation.[16] In contrast with fibrillation potentials, fasciculation potentials are more commonly identified in proximal muscles. As expected, the Awaji Criteria have been found in metaanalytic studies to increase the sensitivity of EMG for ALS by more than 10% and maintained specificity at 100%.[17,18] Modification of the Awaji Criteria to include a probable category has been proposed to further increase sensitivity.[19] Despite these facts, the Awaji Criteria have not been widely adopted by the research community owing to concern over the impact of less stringent diagnostic criteria on findings.

EXPECTED ELECTROMYOGRAPHY FINDINGS FOR DISEASE THAT MIMIC AMYOTROPHIC LATERAL SCLEROSIS

Electrodiagnostic testing can elucidate the various pathologies of weakness and can assist the physician in differentiating anterior horn cell loss from central nervous system disease, demyelinating disorders, plexopathies, and disorders of the neuromuscular junction (**Table 3**). The differential diagnosis for ALS is broadest at the earliest stages when only 1 limb seems to be involved on examination with little to no evidence of upper motor neuron signs as is seen with MMN. Hallmarks of MMN on electrodiagnostic studies include normal sensory responses with motor conduction blocks at nonentrapment sites of 2 or more nerves, demonstrating demyelination as the pathologic basis rather than anterior horn cell loss. Patchy symptoms and electrodiagnostic findings strongly suggest MMN, because this disease affects individual peripheral nerves rather than the diffuse myotomal involvement expected in ALS.[20] Challenges

| Table 2 |
| Awaji Electrodiagnostic Criteria diagnostic categories |

Diagnostic Category	Requirements
Clinically definite ALS	Clinical or electrophysiologic evidence of UMN + LMN signs on clinical examination in 3 body regions
Clinically probable ALS	Clinical or electrophysiologic evidence of UMN + LMN signs on clinical examination in 2 body regions, with some UMN signs rostral to the LMN signs
Clinically possible ALS	Clinical or electrophysiologic evidence of UMN + LMN signs in 1 body region, OR UMN signs in 2 or more body regions, OR LMN signs rostral to UMN signs, AND neuroimaging and clinical laboratory studies will have been performed and other diagnoses must have been excluded

Abbreviations: ALS, amyotrophic lateral sclerosis; body regions, bulbar, cervical, thoracic, lumbosacral; LMN, lower motor neuron; UMN, upper motor neuron.

Data from de Carvalho M, Dengler R, Eisen A, et al. Electrodiagnostic criteria for diagnosis of ALS. Clin Neurophysiol 2008;119(3):497–503.

Table 3
Electrodiagnostic findings in ALS mimics

Disorder	Electrodiagnostic Findings
Multifocal motor neuropathy	Normal SNAPs Conduction block Prolonged latencies Prolonged F-waves Slowed conduction velocities ± Neurogenic MUPs
Myasthenia gravis	Normal SNAPs and CMAPs Unstable MUPs Decrement with Repetitive Stimulation
Cervical/lumbosacral radiculopathy	Normal SNAPs ± Decreased CMAPs Neurogenic MUPs in isolated myotome
Inclusion body myositis	Normal SNAPs and CMAPs ± Increased insertional activity Myopathic MUPs
Chronic inflammatory Demyelinating polyneuropathy	Prolonged latencies Prolonged F-waves ± Neurogenic MUPs
Hereditary spastic paraplegia	Normal SNAPs and CMAPs Normal MUPs
X-linked spinobulbar muscular atrophy (Kennedy's disease)	Abnormal SNAPs

Abbreviations: ALS, amyotrophic lateral sclerosis; CMAP, compound motor action potential; MUPs, motor unit potentials; SNAPs, sensory nerve action potentials.

include identifying proximal conduction block as well as the possibility of MMN without overt conduction block. Needle EMG in MMN may identify increased spontaneous activity with large, polyphasic motor units reflecting secondary axonal damage. Because these needle electrode examination findings in MMN may overlap with those expected in ALS, motor nerve conduction studies may be more useful to distinguish these diagnoses.

Sensory nerve conduction study abnormalities may indicate another common ALS mimic disease. In spinal-bulbar muscular atrophy (Kennedy's disease), pathologic involvement of the dorsal root ganglia commonly results in sensory nerve conduction abnormalities.[21] By contrast, in the absence of a comorbid peripheral polyneuropathy, sensory nerve conduction studies are expected to be normal in ALS.

Neurogenic changes on needle EMG are not unique to ALS, but a diagnosis of ALS is best supported by widespread changes that cannot be explained by another cause. Because the incidence of spinal structural abnormalities increases with an aging population, it is crucial to differentiate cervical and lumbosacral radiculopathies from motor neuron disease. Electrodiagnostic testing in radiculopathies demonstrate normal sensory responses and potentially decreased compound motor action potentials (CMAPs). Needle EMG identifies acute or chronic denervation in a single myotome or multiple myotomes in a polyradiculopathy, as well as in corresponding paraspinals. Bilateral limb involvement is rare. A combination of upper and lower motor neuron signs can be seen in a cervical radiculomyelopathy secondary to cervical spondylosis with nerve root compression resulting in lower motor neuron signs at the level of spondylosis and upper motor neuron signs below it. Monomelic amyotrophy (Hirayama's disease) is characterized by unilateral wasting and weakness in the C7 to T1 myo-tomes and clinically can be concerning for early ALS. The lack of diffuse active dener-vation with chronic reinnervation changes outside of this region on needle EMG differentiates it from ALS.

Bulbar-onset ALS can be clinically challenging to differentiate from myasthenia gravis, specifically myasthenia gravis with muscle-specific kinase antibodies, which can lack oculomotor symptoms.[22] Nerve conduction studies are normal and needle EMG lacks denervation changes that occur in motor neuron disease. The needle EMG may identify unstable motor unit action potentials with small amplitudes and short durations, similar to a myopathic process. Slow repetitive stimulation reveals greater than 10% decrement. However, as mentioned, decrement with repetitive stim-ulation can also be seen in ALS as a result of instability of the neuromuscular transmis-sion in the collateral nerve sprouts.[23]

DIAGNOSTIC LABORATORY AND IMAGING TESTING

There are no set guidelines for laboratory or radiologic testing in the workup of ALS. Testing should be driven by clinical suspicion for alternative diagnoses based on pre-senting symptoms (**Table 4**). Thyrotoxicosis, heavy metal toxicity, and human immu-nodeficiency virus infection can result in both upper and lower motor neuron signs and targeted appropriate laboratory testing should be completed when suspected. Muscle

Table 4
Differential diagnosis and laboratory testing for motor neuron disease

Clinical Presentation	Differential Diagnosis	Diagnostic Testing Recommended
Bulbar-onset	Myasthenia gravis	Acetylcholine receptor and MuSK antibodies
	Brainstem tumor	Brain MRI
Lower motor neuron predominant	Multifocal motor neuropathy	GM1 antibodies
	Spinobulbar muscular atrophy (Kennedy's disease)	Genetic testing
	Spinal muscular atrophy	Genetic testing
	Hypothyroidism	Thyroid-stimulating hormone
	Paraproteinemias	Serum protein electrophoresis/ immunofixation
	Paraneoplastic	Antibody panel (serum, CSF)
	Inclusion body myositis	Muscle biopsy
	Lyme disease/West Nile virus/polio/syphilis	Serology
	Tay-Sachs disease	Hexosaminidase A level
	Heavy metal intoxication	24-h urine collection for heavy metals
Upper motor neuron predominant	Copper deficiency	Serum copper and zinc
	B_{12} deficiency	Vitamin B_{12}, methylmalonic acid, homocysteine
	HIV	HIV
	Tropical Spastic Paraparesis	Human T-cell lymphotropic virus 1 serology
	Adrenomyeloneuropathy	Very long chain fatty acids
	HSP	Genetic testing
	Multiple sclerosis	Brain and spine MRI
Mixed	Spine disease	Spine MRI

Abbreviations: CSF, cerebrospinal fluid; HIV, human immunodeficiency virus; HSP, hereditary spastic paraplegia; MuSK, muscle-specific kinase.

enzyme levels may be slightly elevated in ALS, but values of greater than 2 to 3 times normal should raise suspicion for a myopathic process. Concern for late-onset hexosaminidase A deficiency in the Ashkenazi Jewish population can be addressed with urine enzyme testing. Anti-GM1 antibodies are considered pathogenic for MMN. However, their absence does not exclude diagnosis because it is estimated that only 60% of patients are found to have increased anti-GM1 antibodies.[20] Testing of onconeural antibodies should be considered when there is concern for a paraneoplastic syndrome. Several case reports have identified onconeural antibodies in patients diagnosed with ALS, leading to the discovery of an underlying cancer, but there is no current recommendation for systematic screening.[24]

In individuals with limb weakness without bulbar or respiratory involvement, an MRI of the cervical spine is useful to rule out mixed cord and root compression.[25] MRI of the cervical spine may also be useful in the diagnosis of monomelic amyotrophy because there may be evidence of cord atrophy and displacement of the cord on flexion and extension views.[26] Infiltrative lesions of the tongue and pharynx may be identified on MRI when signs and symptoms are isolated to the bulbar region.[27] T2 hyperintensity of the corticospinal tract can be pronounced in ALS but has low sensitivity and limited specificity. T1 hyperintensity in the anterolateral column of the cervical cord can be observed in patients with ALS.[28] Neuromuscular ultrasound examination is an emerging tool that can identify pathologic changes associated with ALS. These changes may include evidence of decreased nerve cross-sectional areas (which differs from the nerve enlargement findings in demyelinating polyneuropathies), muscular atrophy (as opposed to muscle edema and swelling seen in inflammatory myopathies), and fasciculations when not present clinically or on electrodiagnostic testing.[29]

DNA analysis can confirm a diagnosis of Kennedy's disease (spinobulbar muscular atrophy), which should be considered in individuals with bulbar symptoms and gynecomastia. Consideration for DNA testing should also be given for hereditary spastic paraplegia in individuals with upper motor neuron signs and a slowly progressive paraplegia resulting from spasticity without lower motor neuron involvement. DNA analysis is also useful in those with atypical presentations and a family history of ALS to identify common mutations associated with familial ALS, including SOD1 and C9orf72.

USEFULNESS OF ELECTROMYOGRAPHY FOR PROGNOSTICATION

Clinical monitoring continues to remain the best tool for prognostication. The ALS Functional Rating Score (ALS-FRS), Medical Research Council score, and forced vital capacity are a few tools used clinically and in research to track disease progression. Electrodiagnostic evaluation can provide some insight into disease progression, which can be extrapolated to prognosis. Motor unit number estimates (MUNEs) reflect an estimated number of functional surviving motor neurons. A decrease in MUNEs and mean CMAP amplitudes are most directly correlated to rapid progression and a fatal outcome.[30] MUNE has been studied as an independent predictor of survival in ALS.[31] CMAPs of less than 20% of normal for age indicate severe motor loss.[32] Abnormal repetitive stimulation and single fiber EMG tend to indicate a poorer prognosis.[33] Profound denervation activity in multiple muscles is associated with a shorter median survival time and carries more prognostic value than analysis of motor unit potential morphology.[34]

ELECTRODIAGNOSTIC STUDIES AS BIOMARKERS TO MONITOR PROGRESSION

There is great interest in establishing biomarkers as indicators of subclinical disease activity in ALS, in the hope that these would allow earlier diagnosis as well as more sensitive measures of response to therapeutics. Reliable biomarkers could replace gross endpoints, such as death or initiation of mechanical ventilation, or less sensitive clinical measures currently used in clinical trials, such as the ALS-FRS or Medical Research Council scale. In addition, traditional clinical measures such as these leave room for subjective interpretation. Several electrodiagnostic techniques have been used specifically for tracking disease progression in individuals with ALS, including MUNE, the Motor Unit Nerve Index (MUNIX), the Neurophysiologic Index, and the Cumulative Motor Index. In addition, transcranial magnetic stimulation has been described as an emerging technique to provide insight into upper as well as lower motor neuron function.

MUNE is a quantitative method to assess loss of anterior horn cells and has been used to measure the loss of motor neurons in ALS clinical trials. A variety of MUNE techniques have been described in the literature. The objective of MUNE is to calculate the number of motor units in a muscle by measuring supramaximal CMAP and dividing by the average size of single motor unit potentials. MUNE can identify lower motor neuron loss before weakness and signs on physical examination. The loss of motor units in a muscle as measured by MUNEs is typically rapid initially and then more gradual for the remaining motor units.[32] Although this technique has been available since 1971, it has not been adopted in common clinical practice. One reason for this may be concerns over variability in technique and, therefore, the reliability of the results. Another limiting factor is the time burden for performing MUNE.

MUNIX also provides a quantitative estimate of the number of lower motor neurons supplying a muscle, expressed as the ideal case motor unit count. This is calculated based on the area and power of the CMAP with supramaximal stimulation, and area and power of surface EMG interference pattern at different levels of voluntary contraction. MUNIX scores may be reported for either individual muscles or aggregated scores for a selection of muscles. MUNIX can be performed in 3 to 5 minutes per muscle, which makes it quicker to administer in comparison with MUNE. MUNIX scores typically show greater decline over time as compared with the ALS-FRS, with an average decline of 3.2% per month, regardless of the site of onset of symptoms.[35]

The Neurophysiologic Index is another composite score used to monitor disease progression and it is calculated from the CMAP amplitude, distal motor latency, and F-wave persistence.[36] This measure is attractive as compared with MUNE because it involves commonly performed studies rather than new techniques, is easily obtained during routine studies, and does not require specialized software. This measure has been shown to be more sensitive to change as compared with quantitative measures of muscle strength.

In an effort to further simplify available electrodiagnostic measures, the Cumulative Motor Index has been proposed as a simple electrodiagnostic measure to monitor progression. This measure consists of the sum of the supramaximal CMAP amplitudes of the abductor pollicis brevis, abductor digiti minimi, biceps, tibialis anterior, extensor digitorum brevis, and abductor hallucis. Again, this electrophysiologic measure reveals greater sensitivity to change over time for most individuals with ALS studied as compared with the ALS-FRS.[37]

Transcranial magnetic stimulation provides a means of interrogating both central and peripheral motor nerve conduction and allows an electrodiagnostic glimpse into the function of the upper motor neurons. Recent data suggest that cortical hyperexcitability is among the earliest pathologic changes seen in ALS patients.[38] Although not currently used diagnostically, transcranial motor evoked potentials in ALS have shown abnormalities in threshold, cortical inhibition, latency, and motor control with a normal cortical silence period. Threshold tracking can show changes in axonal membrane excitability.

ELECTROMYOGRAPHY STUDIES TO GUIDE INTERVENTIONS FOR MOTOR NEURON DISEASE

Electrodiagnostic studies allow for the assessment of subclinical disease extent, which may prompt medical intervention. Electrodiagnostic studies of the diaphragm in persons with ALS can reveal respiratory musculature impairment in asymptomatic individuals and, when dysfunction is present, can guide the clinician to implement noninvasive ventilatory support to prolong survival.[39] In addition, these studies provide a mechanism to assess respiratory function in the case of a patient who is unable to complete spirometry owing to facial muscle weakness.[40]

DISCUSSION AND IMPLICATIONS FOR CLINICAL PRACTICE

Although ALS is the most common adult form of motor neuron disease, considerable lags in establishing a diagnosis remain commonplace. These delays, once thought to be inconsequential owing to the lack of therapeutics for this disease, now have more significant ramifications by limiting access to early initiation of disease-modifying treatments and interventions that may slow disease progression or enhance quality of life. The Awaji Electrodiagnostic Criteria were proposed to increase the sensitivity of EMG for diagnosis of ALS while maintaining high specificity. Although the Awaji Diagnostic Criteria have not yet been widely accepted in the research community, they may be of benefit in clinical practice to expedite diagnosis.

The identification of ALS mimic disorders is paramount to screen for potentially treatable causes of disease, most of which confer a more favorable prognosis. A careful history and physical examination is essential for guiding an appropriate diagnostic evaluation to assess for these conditions. Among available electrodiagnostic techniques, sensory and motor nerve conduction studies and needle electrode examination add the most value to identify common ALS mimic diseases.

By identifying subclinical disease involvement, electrodiagnostic abnormalities may guide patient management by foreshadowing clinical weakness, disease progression, and prognosis. CMAP amplitudes reflect the survival of motor neurons and can provide a quantitative assessment of disease severity in a specific muscle. Respiratory muscle abnormalities by needle EMG may prompt providers to expedite further neuromuscular respiratory assessment and treatment interventions. The information gleaned by EMG studies has the potential to be of great use to the interdisciplinary ALS care team in providing education, counseling, and timely interventions to maximize function of individuals with ALS.

As new pharmacologic therapies emerge for ALS, many questions remain about the best tools to monitor individual patient response to treatment. Traditional outcome measures for ALS trials are limited by their subjective nature and lack of sensitivity to change. Although not widely used in clinical practice, specialized electrodiagnostic techniques, such as MUNE, MUNIX, the Neurophysiologic Index, and the Cumulative Motor Index, may be useful to monitor subclinical disease progression and may serve to provide ongoing monitoring of effect for both research or clinical settings.

SUMMARY

Although electrodiagnostic studies are often thought of as yielding only a binary conclusion—either positive or negative for the diagnosis of ALS—there is ample evidence to suggest greater clinical usefulness for patient management. Attention should be paid to the detailed findings of nerve conduction studies and needle electrode examination to maximize the value of this tool for clinical management.

REFERENCES

1. Mehta P, Kaye W, Bryan L, et al. Prevalence of amyotrophic lateral sclerosis - United States, 2012-2013. MMWR Surveill Summ 2016;65(8):1–12.
2. Burrell JR, Vucic S, Kiernan MC. Isolated bulbar phenotype of amyotrophic lateral sclerosis. Amyotroph Lateral Scler 2011;12(4):283–9.
3. Chio A, Calvo A, Moglia C, et al. Phenotypic heterogeneity of amyotrophic lateral sclerosis: a population based study. J Neurol Neurosurg Psychiatry 2011;82(7): 740–6.
4. Ravits J, Appel S, Baloh RH, et al. Deciphering amyotrophic lateral sclerosis: what phenotype, neuropathology and genetics are telling us about pathogenesis. Amyotroph Lateral Scler Frontotemporal Degener 2013;14(Suppl 1):5–18.
5. Swinnen B, Robberecht W. The phenotypic variability of amyotrophic lateral sclerosis. Nat Rev Neurol 2014;10(11):661–70.
6. Wolf J, Safer A, Wöhrle JC, et al. Variability and prognostic relevance of different phenotypes in amyotrophic lateral sclerosis - data from a population-based registry. J Neurol Sci 2014;345(1–2):164–7.
7. Mitchell JD, Callagher P, Gardham J, et al. Timelines in the diagnostic evaluation of people with suspected amyotrophic lateral sclerosis (ALS)/motor neuron disease (MND)–a 20-year review: can we do better? Amyotroph Lateral Scler 2010;11(6):537–41.
8. Woolley SC, Jonathan SK. Cognitive and behavioral impairment in amyotrophic lateral sclerosis. Phys Med Rehabil Clin N Am 2008;19(3):607–17, xi.
9. Chio A, Mora G, Lauria G. Pain in amyotrophic lateral sclerosis. Lancet Neurol 2017;16(2):144–57.
10. Paganoni S, Macklin EA, Lee A, et al. Diagnostic timelines and delays in diagnosing amyotrophic lateral sclerosis (ALS). Amyotroph Lateral Scler Frontotemporal Degener 2014;15(5–6):453–6.
11. Hatanaka Y, Higashihara M, Chiba T, et al. Utility of repetitive nerve stimulation test for ALS diagnosis. Clin Neurophysiol 2017;128(5):823–9.
12. Zheng C, Zhu D, Lu F, et al. Compound muscle action potential decrement to repetitive nerve stimulation between Hirayama disease and amyotrophic lateral sclerosis. J Clin Neurophysiol 2017;34(2):119–25.
13. Babu S, Pioro EP, Li J, et al. Optimizing muscle selection for electromyography in amyotrophic lateral sclerosis. Muscle Nerve 2017;56(1):36–44.
14. Brooks BR, Miller RG, Swash M, et al. El Escorial revisited: revised criteria for the diagnosis of amyotrophic lateral sclerosis. Amyotroph Lateral Scler Other Motor Neuron Disord 2000;1(5):293–9.
15. Traynor BJ, Codd MB, Corr B, et al. Clinical features of amyotrophic lateral sclerosis according to the El Escorial and Airlie House diagnostic criteria: a population-based study. Arch Neurol 2000;57(8):1171–6.
16. de Carvalho M, Dengler R, Eisen A, et al. Electrodiagnostic criteria for diagnosis of ALS. Clin Neurophysiol 2008;119(3):497–503.
17. Jang JS, Bae JS. AWAJI criteria are not always superior to the previous criteria: a meta-analysis. Muscle Nerve 2015;51(6):822–9.
18. Geevasinga N, Menon P, Scherman DB, et al. Diagnostic criteria in amyotrophic lateral sclerosis: a multicenter prospective study. Neurology 2016;87(7):684–90.

19. Geevasinga N, Loy CT, Menon P, et al. Awaji criteria improves the diagnostic sensitivity in amyotrophic lateral sclerosis: a systematic review using individual patient data. Clin Neurophysiol 2016;127(7):2684–91.

20. Muley SA, Parry GJ. Multifocal motor neuropathy. J Clin Neurosci 2012;19(9): 1201–9.

21. Ferrante MA, Wilbourn AJ. The characteristic electrodiagnostic features of Kennedy's disease. Muscle Nerve 1997;20(3):323–9.

22. Huijbers MG, Niks EH, Klooster R, et al. Myasthenia gravis with muscle specific kinase antibodies mimicking amyotrophic lateral sclerosis. Neuromuscul Disord 2016;26(6):350–3.

23. Rocha JA, Reis C, Simões F, et al. Diagnostic investigation and multidisciplinary management in motor neuron disease. J Neurol 2005;252(12):1435–47.

24. Corcia P, Gordon PH, Camdessanche JP. Is there a paraneoplastic ALS? Amyotroph Lateral Scler Frontotemporal Degener 2015;16(3–4):252–7.

25. Lenglet T, Camdessanche JP. Amyotrophic lateral sclerosis or not: keys for the diagnosis. Rev Neurol (Paris) 2017;173(5):280–7.

26. Rowland LP. Diagnosis of amyotrophic lateral sclerosis. J Neurol Sci 1998; 160(Suppl 1):S6–24.

27. Wood-Allum C, Shaw PJ. Motor neurone disease: a practical update on diagnosis and management. Clin Med (Lond) 2010;10(3):252–8.

28. Turner MR, Kiernan MC, Leigh PN, et al. Biomarkers in amyotrophic lateral sclerosis. Lancet Neurol 2009;8(1):94–109.

29. Cartwright MS, Walker FO, Griffin LP, et al. Peripheral nerve and muscle ultrasound in amyotrophic lateral sclerosis. Muscle Nerve 2011;44(3):346–51.

30. Liu XX, Zhang J, Zheng JY, et al. Stratifying disease stages with different progression rates determined by electrophysiological tests in patients with amyotrophic lateral sclerosis. Muscle Nerve 2009;39(3):304–9.

31. Armon C, Brandstater ME. Motor unit number estimate-based rates of progression of ALS predict patient survival. Muscle Nerve 1999;22(11):1571–5.

32. Daube JR. Electrodiagnostic studies in amyotrophic lateral sclerosis and other motor neuron disorders. Muscle Nerve 2000;23(10):1488–502.

33. Kimura J. Electrodiagnosis in diseases of nerve and muscle: principles and practice. Oxford: Oxford University Press; 2000.

34. Krarup C. Lower motor neuron involvement examined by quantitative electromyography in amyotrophic lateral sclerosis. Clin Neurophysiol 2011;122(2):414–22.

35. Neuwirth C, Barkhaus PE, Burkhardt C, et al. Tracking motor neuron loss in a set of six muscles in amyotrophic lateral sclerosis using the Motor Unit Number Index (MUNIX): a 15-month longitudinal multicentre trial. J Neurol Neurosurg Psychiatry 2015;86(11):1172–9.

36. Swash M, de Carvalho M. The neurophysiological index in ALS. Amyotroph Lateral Scler Other Mot Neuron Disord 2004;5(Suppl 1):108–10.

37. Nandedkar SD, Barkhaus PE, Stalberg EV. Cumulative motor index: an index to study progression of amyotrophic lateral sclerosis. J Clin Neurophysiol 2015; 32(1):79–85.

38. Vucic S, Kiernan MC. Transcranial magnetic stimulation for the assessment of neurodegenerative disease. Neurotherapeutics 2017;14(1):91–106.

39. Stewart H, Eisen A, Road J, et al. Electromyography of respiratory muscles in amyotrophic lateral sclerosis. J Neurol Sci 2001;191(1–2):67–73.

40. Eisen A, Swash M. Clinical neurophysiology of ALS. Clin Neurophysiol 2001; 112(12):2190–201.

The Value of Electrodiagnostic Studies in Predicting Treatment Outcomes for Patients with Spine Pathologies

Kevin Barrette, MD[a],*, Joshua Levin, MD[b], Derek Miles, DPT[c], David J. Kennedy, MD[d]

KEYWORDS

- Electromyography • Radiculopathy • Diagnosis • Outcome • Spine • Low back pain
- Epidural steroid injection • Therapy

KEY POINTS

- Electrodiagnostics have a high specificity, but a low sensitivity for radiculopathy.
- In certain cases, electrodiagnostics can be a valuable tool to aid in the diagnostic algorithm.
- The diagnostic confidence in the test results are predicated on the prevalence of the suspected pathology.

INTRODUCTION

Spine pathology represents a major public health concern, with estimates showing prevalence of 70% to 90% of adults experiencing these maladies at some point in their lives.[1,2] The number of patient visits related to spine pain has continually increased, as has the number of opioid prescriptions written for them and the number of referrals to specialists.[3] For the subset of patients with radicular pain, studies have shown benefit from several different treatments, including physical therapy (PT),[4,5] epidural steroid injections (ESIs),[6–12] and surgical interventions.

Disclosures: The authors have no relevant financial disclosures.
[a] Department of Orthopedics, Stanford University, 450 Broadway, Redwood City, CA 94063, USA; [b] Department of Orthopedics and Neurosurgery, Stanford University, 213 Quarry Road, Palo Alto, CA 94304, USA; [c] Department of Rehabilitation, Stanford Children's Hospital, 725 Welch Road, Palo Alto, CA 94304, USA; [d] Department of Physical Medicine and Rehabilitation, Vanderbilt University Medical Center, 2201 Children's Way, Nashville, TN 37212, USA
* Corresponding author. PM&R, 450 Broadway Street, Pavillion C MC/6342, Redwood City, CA 94063.
E-mail address: kevinfbarrette@gmail.com

Phys Med Rehabil Clin N Am 29 (2018) 681–687
https://doi.org/10.1016/j.pmr.2018.06.004
1047-9651/18/Published by Elsevier Inc.

Given current public health trends, better management strategies for back pain are necessary, but with the wide array of interventions available, it is often difficult to predict individual patient response to treatment. This dilemma is confounded by the lack of a single gold standard for the diagnosis of radiculopathy. The diagnosis of radiculopathy is generally made based on clinical impression gathered from the history and physical. This can become problematic, as multiple non–spine pain generators have been shown to radiate in the arm[13] or leg,[14,15] which could mimic radicular pain. Use of imaging is often problematic because of the high number of asymptomatic abnormals. Electrodiagnostic testing often adds useful information to help reach a diagnosis.[13–19]

Electrodiagnostics (EDX) are physiologic tests for assessing radiculopathies, and the electromyography (EMG) portion is the single most important technique for assessing denervation.[19,20] EDX may provide valuable information regarding both the localization and the presence of axonal nerve damage at the nerve root. EDX can also help evaluate for other conditions that can mimic radiculopathy[21]

EDX for radiculopathy represents a high specificity, low sensitivity test.[22] Thus, it serves as a good way to confirm a diagnosis, but is not a good screening test due to the low sensitivity. However, the question does arise, could EDX be useful in predicting which patients might respond better to a given treatment plan? This article explores current evidence for the predictive value of EDX for the effectiveness of PT, ESIs, and surgery in patients with cervical and lumbosacral radiculopathy. Then, those data are used to give examples of when EDX testing may be of clinical utility based on disease prevalence and the diagnostic confidence of a given test combined with current treatment paradigms.

PHYSICAL THERAPY AND OTHER CONSERVATIVE CARE

Only one study to date has evaluated the utility of EDX to predict outcomes from physical therapy. Savage and colleagues[23] studied patients with "sciatica" who underwent EDX performed by a physical therapist. One weakness of the study is that the criteria for a positive EMG was denervation in limb muscles and/or isolated abnormal findings in the paraspinal muscles. Diagnosing radiculopathy by paraspinal abnormality alone is not a standard EDX criterion for radiculopathy.[24] Despite this, patients who met the EMG criteria for radiculopathy demonstrated better improvement in low back–related disability outcomes after physical therapy compared with those with normal EDX.[23] There has not been a study on EDX predicting response to chiropractic care, acupuncture, massage, or oral medications. This may be because of the relatively little evidence for benefit of these conditions for radiculopathy.[25]

EPIDURAL STEROID INJECTIONS

The role of EDX in predicting response to ESIs has been studied more extensively than its role in predicting outcomes from other treatments.

Fish and colleagues[26] retrospectively studied the predictive value of EDX on outcomes from lumbar transforaminal ESIs performed on 39 patients. EDX were deemed positive based on findings of denervation and/or reinnervation. In this small study, the investigators showed a slightly greater improvement in Oswestry Disability Index in the EMG-positive group, no difference was seen in pain scores between the EMG-positive (18 patients) and EMG-negative (21 patients) groups.

Marchetti and colleagues[27] retrospectively studied the predictive value of EMG in patients with mixed diagnoses who received an ESI (either transforaminal, interlaminar, or caudal). EMG findings were considered positive based on denervation or reinnervation. They found no significant differences in leg and back pain improvements between patients who had positive, negative, or equivocal EMG findings. The investigators concluded from this study that normal EMG findings should not preclude patients from receiving ESI.

Cosgrove and colleagues[28] studied the response to interlaminar ESI in patients with spinal stenosis. No correlation was seen between EDX findings and outcomes; however, only 1 of the 16 patients in this study met the EDX criteria for radiculopathy (denervation), so very limited information can be drawn from this study.

Annaswamy and colleagues[29] prospectively studied 89 subjects with mixed diagnoses who received lumbar interlaminar ESIs. EDX were deemed positive based on findings of denervation, and an abnormal EMG was defined as those with either positive or equivocal EMG findings. The investigators found that an abnormal EMG better predicted improvement in both pain and functional scores; however, both groups showed minimal clinically relevant mean improvements in Visual Analog Scale pain scores (approximately 2 in the abnormal EMG group and 1 in the normal EMG group).

McCormick and colleagues[30] studied 170 subjects with either chronic lumbar (148) or cervical (22) radicular pain in a hybrid study design. EMG findings were considered abnormal based on denervation and/or reinnervation; however, those who had denervation were analyzed separately. The investigators found that patients with lumbar radiculopathy with abnormal EDX were more likely to have better intermediate and long-term outcomes compared with those without abnormal EDX. Additionally, no differences were seen when comparing patients who had denervation with those without denervation on EDX. EDX did not predict outcomes in patients with cervical radicular pain. The investigators concluded that EMG is a predictor of long-term outcomes after lumbar transforaminal ESI, but felt the numbers were too small in the cervical spine to draw clear conclusions.[30]

All of these studies must be placed into appropriate context given that the EDX testing was generally done at the discretion of the treating physician, which may induce a selection bias. Additionally, the criteria for calling a positive EDX examination also varied between studies, which also introduces a level of imprecision. Last, in contrast to a transforaminal epidural steroid injection, some of the interventional treatments used in these studies have been shown to not be effective (such as caudal or non–image-guided ESI),[11,31] even if done for the appropriate indication of radiculopathy.

SPINE SURGERY

The literature for EDX in patients undergoing surgical interventions is also somewhat limited. Tullberg and colleagues[32] studied EDX in 20 patients undergoing surgery for lumbosacral radicular pain from a disk herniation. The EDX consisted of needle EMG (it was considered abnormal if there were abnormalities, either abnormal spontaneous activity or recruitment/morphology changes, in one muscle), F-wave analysis, and somatosensory evoked potentials. Patients with normal preoperative EDX had significantly worse outcomes compared with those with an abnormality in at least 1 of the 3 sections of the EDX analsysis.[32]

Alrawi and colleagues[33] prospectively studied 20 patients treated with anterior cervical interbody fusion. The 8 patients with electrodiagnostic evidence of radiculopathy, defined as abnormal spontaneous activity and long duration, polyphasic motor unit action potentials, had better surgical outcomes than those without abnormal EDX.

DISCUSSION

To be useful, the previous data must be placed into appropriate context. First, there is a general trend in the literature showing that those with EDX-confirmed radiculopathy do better with the treatments than those with negative EDX testing. At first glance this is somewhat paradoxic, in which those with physiologic evidence of nerve damage do better than those without evidence of damage. It is not likely that corticosteroids, physical therapy, or even surgery actually fixes confirmed axonal damage. Instead, it is more likely that EDX increases the precision of the diagnosis and the subsequent homogeneity of study participants, thus enhancing the outcomes.

The role of electrodiagnosis in patients with radiculopathy is generally to increase the precision of diagnosis. These studies provide valuable information about the root levels involved, and whether the denervation is more acute or chronic. If other peripheral nerve disorders are on the differential diagnosis for a particular patient, this can be another way that the study adds value. This information should then be used to guide subsequent clinical management. As in other conditions, the additional information that electrodiagnosis adds to the clinical management of radiculopathy varies. To make appropriate utilization decisions, the practitioner must understand both the diagnostic confidence of the EDX results and the treatment options available.

DIAGNOSTIC CONFIDENCE OF A TEST

To understand the utility of information gleamed from a diagnostic test, the sensitivity and specificity of the test for the condition being analyzed should be considered. This is calculated using a 2 × 2 table, as shown in **Fig. 1**. Although a full discussion regarding sensitivity and specificity of EDX testing is beyond the scope of this article, the sensitivity and specificity of EDX testing varies based on the underlying pathology and the exact combination of tests used. Typical factors that affect the sensitivity and specificity of electrodiagnostic studies for radiculopathy include the number of muscles tested for radiculopathy,[24,34,35] among others.

Although important, the sensitivity and specificity of a given test for a given condition are only part of the story. The other consideration that must be accounted for is the prevalence of a condition. Similar to sensitivity and specificity, the prevalence of different pathologies can vary significantly. Many factors affect the prevalence of pathology in a population, including but not limited to the presenting symptoms, patient demographics, and clinic referral patterns.[36,37] When the prevalence of a condition is combined with the sensitivity and specificity of a test, the diagnostic confidence can be calculated (**Fig. 2**). Diagnostic confidence represents the odds that the results of the test are true based on disease prevalence and the sensitivity and specificity of the test. A couple of examples will help clarify the role of prevalence in the diagnostic confidence, as well help demonstrate when EDX testing may add clinically useful information.

Test	Disease (Gold standard)	
	Positive	Negative
Positive	a	b
Negative	c	d

Fig. 1. A 2 × 2 table outlining sensitivity and specificity based on a gold standard. a = true positive, b = false positive, c = false negative, d = true negative. Sensitive = a/a + c (true positive/true positive + false negative). Specificity = d/b + d (true negative/false positive + true negative).

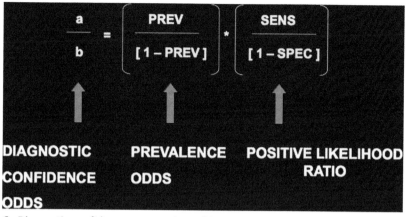

Fig. 2. Diagnostic confidence expressed as odds is a combination of prevalence odds and positive likelihood ratio (which is calculated based on the sensitivity and specificity of the test).

Example 1. A 30-year-old patient with 4-week history of abrupt-onset, lancinating right leg pain in an L5 distribution and weakness in the extensor hallucis longus. Magnetic resonance scan shows a far lateral L5/S1 disk extrusion affecting the right L5 nerve root. For patients in this age group, with this combination of symptoms, signs, and imaging findings, the prevalence of lumbar radicular pain is high, and other pathologies would be exceedingly rare. The diagnostic confidence is high given the history, physical, and MRI findings. In such a scenario, a negative or positive EDX examination will not likely change the suspected clinical diagnosis, as a negative test does not rule out the condition, given the relatively low sensitivity of needle EMG to detect radiculopathy, and a positive test merely confirms what is already known.

Example 2. A 45-year-old patient with a many-year history of diffuse neck pain, and a 4-month history of right hand and forearm numbness that is worse with repetitive activities and at night. In this scenario there would be ambiguity in the potential diagnosis, with 2 primary considerations in the differential diagnosis: carpal tunnel syndrome or cervical radicular pain. Either of these pathologies could easily result in the reported symptoms. Both have a relatively high prevalence in a population with these symptoms. The results of EDX testing may significantly alter treatment recommendations.

SUMMARY

Electrodiagnostic testing is a powerful tool that when appropriately used can aide in the evaluation and management of patients with suspected radiculopathies. To appropriately use this test, the practitioner must consider the disease prevalence combined with the sensitivity and specificity of the test. Additionally, the practitioner should consider if the results of the testing would change the treatment paradigm. Only if the results of the EDX testing actually changes or offers sufficient insights into the proposed diagnosis or treatment recommendations should it be undertaken.

REFERENCES

1. Freburger JK, Holmes GM, Agans RP, et al. The rising prevalence of chronic low back pain. Arch Intern Med 2009;169(3):251–8.

2. Deyo RA, Mirza SK, Martin BI. Back pain prevalence and visit rates: estimates from U.S. national surveys, 2002. Spine 2006;31(23):2724–7.

3. Mafi JN, McCarthy EP, Davis RB, et al. Worsening trends in the management and treatment of back pain. JAMA Intern Med 2013;173(17):1573–81.

4. Hahne AJ, Ford JJ, Hinman RS, et al. Outcomes and adverse events from physiotherapy functional restoration for lumbar disc herniation with associated radiculopathy. Disabil Rehabil 2011;33(17–18):1537–47.

5. Hahne AJ, Ford JJ, McMeeken JM. Conservative management of lumbar disc herniation with associated radiculopathy: a systematic review. Spine 2010; 35(11):E488–504.

6. Roberts ST, Willick SE, Rho ME, et al. Efficacy of lumbosacral transforaminal epidural steroid injections: a systematic review. PM R 2009;1(7):657–68.

7. Abdi S, Datta S, Trescot AM, et al. Epidural steroids in the management of chronic spinal pain: a systematic review. Pain Physician 2007;10(1):185–212.

8. Boswell MV, Hansen HC, Trescot AM, et al. Epidural steroids in the management of chronic spinal pain and radiculopathy. Pain Physician 2003;6(3):319–34.

9. MacVicar J, King W, Landers MH, et al. The effectiveness of lumbar transforaminal injection of steroids: a comprehensive review with systematic analysis of the published data. Pain Med 2013;14(1):14–28.

10. Ghahreman A, Ferch R, Bogduk N. The efficacy of transforaminal injection of steroids for the treatment of lumbar radicular pain. Pain Med 2010;11(8):1149–68.

11. Mattie R, McCormick Z, Yu S, et al. Are all epidurals created equally? A systematic review of the literature on caudal, interlaminar, and transforaminal injections from the last 5 years. Curr Phys Med Rehabil Rep 2015;3(2):159–72.

12. Sharma AK, Vorobeychik Y, Wasserman R, et al. The effectiveness and risks of fluoroscopically guided lumbar interlaminar epidural steroid injections: a systematic review with comprehensive analysis of the published data. Pain Med 2017; 18(2):239–51.

13. Kennedy DJ, Mattie R, Nguyen Q, et al. Glenohumeral joint pain referral patterns: a descriptive study. Pain Med 2015;16(8):1603–9.

14. Dreyfuss P, Michaelsen M, Pauza K, et al. The value of medical history and physical examination in diagnosing sacroiliac joint pain. Spine 1996;21(22):2594–602.

15. Lesher JM, Dreyfuss P, Hager N, et al. Hip joint pain referral patterns: a descriptive study. Pain Med 2008;9(1):22–5.

16. Smuck M, Demirjian R, Kennedy DJ. Cervical foraminal versus interlaminar epidurals: risks, benefits, and alternatives. Curr Phys Med Rehabil Rep 2013;1(2): 125–34.

17. Van Zundert J, Huntoon M, Patijn J, et al. 4. Cervical radicular pain. Pain Pract 2010;10(1):1–17.

18. Kreiner DS, Hwang SW, Easa JE, et al. An evidence-based clinical guideline for the diagnosis and treatment of lumbar disc herniation with radiculopathy. Spine J 2014;14(1):180–91.

19. Aminoff MJ, Goodin DS, Parry GJ, et al. Electrophysiologic evaluation of lumbosacral radiculopathies: electromyography, late responses, and somatosensory evoked potentials. Neurology 1985;35(10):1514–8.

20. Annaswamy TM, Bierner SM, Avraham R. Role of electrodiagnosis in patients being considered for epidural steroid injections. PM R 2013;5(5 Suppl):S96–9.

21. Albeck MJ, Taher G, Lauritzen M, et al. Diagnostic value of electrophysiological tests in patients with sciatica. Acta Neurol Scand 2000;101(4):249–54.

22. Cho SC, Ferrante MA, Levin KH, et al. Utility of electrodiagnostic testing in evaluating patients with lumbosacral radiculopathy: an evidence-based review. Muscle Nerve 2010;42(2):276–82.

23. Savage NJ, Fritz JM, Kircher JC, et al. The prognostic value of electrodiagnostic testing in patients with sciatica receiving physical therapy. Eur Spine J 2015; 24(3):434–43.

24. Dillingham TR, Lauder TD, Andary M, et al. Identifying lumbosacral radiculopathies: an optimal electromyographic screen. Am J Phys Med Rehabil 2000; 79(6):496–503.

25. Chou R, Deyo R, Friedly J, et al. Noninvasive treatments for low back pain. Rockville (MD): Agency for Healthcare Research and Quality (US); 2016. Available at: http://www.ncbi.nlm.nih.gov/books/NBK350276/. Accessed November 11, 2016.

26. Fish DE, Shirazi EP, Pham Q. The use of electromyography to predict functional outcome following transforaminal epidural spinal injections for lumbar radiculopathy. J Pain 2008;9(1):64–70.

27. Marchetti J, Verma-Kurvari S, Patel N, et al. Are electrodiagnostic study findings related to a patient's response to epidural steroid injection? PM R 2010;2(11): 1016–20.

28. Cosgrove JL, Bertolet M, Chase SL, et al. Epidural steroid injections in the treatment of lumbar spinal stenosis efficacy and predictability of successful response. Am J Phys Med Rehabil 2011;90(12):1050–5.

29. Annaswamy TM, Bierner SM, Chouteau W, et al. Needle electromyography predicts outcome after lumbar epidural steroid injection. Muscle Nerve 2012;45(3): 346–55.

30. McCormick Z, Cushman D, Caldwell M, et al. Does electrodiagnostic confirmation of radiculopathy predict pain reduction after transforaminal epidural steroid injection? A multicenter study. J Nat Sci 2015;1(8) [pii:e140].

31. Vorobeychik Y, Sharma A, Smith CC, et al. The effectiveness and risks of non-image-guided lumbar interlaminar epidural steroid injections: a systematic review with comprehensive analysis of the published data. Pain Med 2016;17(12): 2185–202.

32. Tullberg T, Svanborg E, Isaccsson J, et al. A preoperative and postoperative study of the accuracy and value of electrodiagnosis in patients with lumbosacral disc herniation. Spine 1993;18(7):837–42.

33. Alrawi MF, Khalil NM, Mitchell P, et al. The value of neurophysiological and imaging studies in predicting outcome in the surgical treatment of cervical radiculopathy. Eur Spine J 2007;16(4):495–500.

34. Dillingham TR, Lauder TD, Andary M, et al. Identification of cervical radiculopathies: optimizing the electromyographic screen. Am J Phys Med Rehabil 2001; 80(2):84–91.

35. Robinson LR, Strakowski J, Kennedy DJ. Is the combined sensory (Robinson) index routinely indicated for all cases of suspected carpal tunnel syndrome undergoing electrodiagnostic evaluation? PM&R 2013;5(5):433–7.

36. DePalma MJ, Ketchum JM, Saullo T. What is the source of chronic low back pain and does age play a role? Pain Med 2011;12(2):224–33.

37. DePalma MJ, Ketchum JM, Saullo TR. Multivariable analyses of the relationships between age, gender, and body mass index and the source of chronic low back pain. Pain Med 2012;13(4):498–506.

Planning Interventions to Treat Brachial Plexopathies

Aaron E. Bunnell, MD[a],*, Dennis S. Kao, MD[b]

KEYWORDS

- Brachial plexus injury • Brachial plexopathy • Nerve transfer • Nerve repair
- Nerve root avulsion • Donor nerve • Neurotization

KEY POINTS

- Electrodiagnosis plays a key role in establishing the location of injury and prognosis in brachial plexus injury.
- Nerve transfer surgery can greatly improve functional outcomes in patients with severe brachial plexus injury.
- Nerve transfer surgery to repair brachial plexus injury is time sensitive and should occur within 3 to 6 months.
- Preoperative electrodiagnostic evaluation of potential donor nerves should be conducted to assess their viability for nerve transfer.

INTRODUCTION

Brachial plexus injury can profoundly affect patient physical function and quality of life.[1] Approximately 1.2% of polytrauma patients suffer brachial plexus injury, with the incidence of injury approaching 5% in motorcycle collisions.[2] Injury is more frequent in males than females, and because injury tends to occur in younger populations, it can have devastating, lifelong effects.

The diagnosis and management of these injuries challenge the individual practitioner and the health care system. Frequently injury is further complicated by comorbid traumatic brain injury, cervical spine injury, and orthopedic injuries.[2,3] Patients with brachial plexus injury require careful coordination of care and a multidisciplinary approach including surgical, electrodiagnostic, pain management, psychological, rehabilitation, and physical and occupational therapy expertise. Fortunately, new surgical options are available to improve functional outcomes. However, these interventions are time dependent, and the window of opportunity is missed if the patient is lost to follow-up.

Disclosure of Conflicts of Interest: None of the authors have any conflicts of interest to disclose.
[a] Department of Rehabilitation Medicine, University of Washington, Box 359740, 325 9th Avenue S, Seattle, WA 98104, USA; [b] Department of Plastic Surgery, University of Washington, 325 9th Avenue S, Seattle, WA 98104, USA
* Corresponding author.
E-mail address: bunnell@uw.edu

The electrodiagnostician serves an important role in the successful management of brachial plexus injury. This starts with diagnosing location and severity of the brachial plexus structures injured and providing prognostic information to the patient and referring physician. In cases where nerve transfer is necessary to restore function, the electrodiagnostician will evaluate the viability of potential donor nerves. Additionally, the electrodiagnostic clinic acts as a key contact point to ensure that the patient has a clear understanding of the required follow-up and that the health care system is appropriately implementing a treatment plan.

ELECTRODIAGNOSTIC ASSESSMENT OF THE BRACHIAL PLEXUS

Because of the complexity of the brachial plexus, there is no single study that can fully evaluate and characterize the nature of injury. The evaluation of brachial plexus injury requires a detailed understanding of the anatomy and its correlation to a complement of sensory and motor nerve conduction studies and needle electromyography (EMG). Each of study contributes specific information regarding the brachial plexus structures injured, the pathophysiology of the lesion, and the prognosis. Most importantly, when compared with other diagnostic studies such as MRI, the electrodiagnostic study provides information about the function of the brachial plexus structures.

Anatomy

The brachial plexus is a complex of peripheral nerves arising from the spinal cord and supplying most of the terminal branches of the upper extremity and shoulder. It is divided into roots, trunks, divisions, cords, and branches.

The roots arise from the spinal nerves C5 through T1 and are comprised of dorsal and ventral rootlets, mixed spinal nerves, anterior and posterior primary rami, and mixed spinal nerve. Anomalies in the brachial plexus are not infrequent—with the plexus predominantly formed from the C4–C7 roots (prefixed) or alternatively from the C6– T2 roots (postfixed).[4] The cervical paraspinals arise from the posterior primary ramus and are important for diagnosing root avulsion. The anterior rami of the roots give off the long thoracic (C5–C7) and the dorsal scapular nerves (C5).

The anterior rami of the roots then form the 3 trunks, with C5 and C6 forming the upper trunk, C7 forming the middle trunk, and C8 and T1 forming the lower trunk. The suprascapular nerve comes off the trunk immediately after the joining of the C5 and C6 roots. The nerve to the subclavius muscle also arises here, but is not clinically important.

Each trunk then divides into an anterior and posterior division (for a total of 6 divisions: 3 posterior and 3 anterior). The anterior and posterior divisions lie posterior to the clavicle and do not usually give off branches.

The divisions subsequently form the cords that are located distal to the clavicle in the axilla. The 3 posterior divisions combine to form the posterior cord and subsequently give off the thoracodorsal, lower and upper subscapular, and axillary and radial nerves. The anterior divisions of the upper and middle trunks combine to form the lateral cord and give off the lateral pectoral, musculocutaneous, and lateral head of the median nerve. The lower trunk anterior division becomes the medial cord and gives off the media brachial cutaneous, medial antebrachial cutaneous, and ulnar nerves and contributes to the medial head of the median nerve.

Timing of Electrodiagnostic Evaluation

The timing of electrodiagnostic evaluation is essential, and the electrodiagnostician must have detailed knowledge of the expected changes over time in needle EMG and nerve conduction findings and interpret these findings based on the duration since injury.

Initial evaluation

An initial evaluation serves to establish the diagnosis of brachial plexopathy, rule out other nerve injury, and provide initial prognostic information. This study is conducted at least 4 weeks after injury, which is sufficient time to observe fibrillation potentials and positive sharp waves in denervated muscle, as well as expected changes in motor and sensory nerve conduction studies. Studies done earlier may result in a false-negative study.

It is useful to conduct a follow-up electrodiagnostic study at approximately 3 to 4 months after injury. The purpose of this study is to evaluate for interval recovery, refine prognosis, and if indicated assess for viable donor nerves. At this time, neuropraxic lesions should demonstrate significant recovery. Because the ideal surgical window occurs at 3 to 6 months, delay in follow-up studies can result in worse outcomes for patient requiring intervention.

At some sites, electrodiagnosis is also completed months after surgery to evaluate for successful reinnervation. In cases in which an extended time period has occurred without clinical or electrodiagnostic recovery, the surgical team may consider late interventions such as arthrodesis, tendon transfer, or functioning free muscle transplantation (FFMT.)

Electrodiagnostic Measures Useful for Evaluation of Brachial Plexus Injury

Compound motor action potential amplitude

The compound motor unit action potential amplitude (CMAP) correlates with the number of motor units functioning within a terminal nerve and provides an estimate the number of axons lost in a brachial plexus injury. The practitioner examines each element of the plexus by choosing the corresponding motor nerve domain[5–7] (**Table 1**). For example, the motor study of the ulnar nerve to ADM will provide information on the integrity of the C8, T1 roots, lower trunk, anterior division, medial cord, and ulnar nerve.

In most of these studies, stimulation occurs distal to the lesion and therefore detects axonal loss rather than demyelination. CMAP amplitude is the most important parameter evaluated. In axonal lesions, Wallerian degeneration will cause the distal CMAP amplitude to decrease by day 2 to 3, with maximal decrease by day 7. Studies done before day 7 may therefore underestimate the extent of axonal loss and the severity of injury. Comparison of the affected side's CMAP amplitude to the contralateral side provides an estimate of the percentage of axons lost (assuming an intact

Table 1				
Motor nerve conduction studies				
Study	**Root**	**Trunk**	**Division**	**Cord**
Ax → deltoid	C5, C6	Upper	Posterior	Posterior
Msc → biceps	C5, C6	Upper	Anterior	Lateral
Radial → EDC	C7, C8	Middle/lower	Posterior	Posterior
Radial → EIP	C7, C8	Middle/lower	Posterior	Posterior
Median → APB	C8, T1	Lower	Anterior	Medial
Ulnar → ADM	C8, T1	Lower	Anterior	Medial
Ulnar → FDI	C8, T1	Lower	Anterior	Medial

contralateral side). Absent or very low amplitudes likely indicate worse prognosis, and intact or mildly affected amplitudes likely indicate better prognosis. However, extensive outcome evidence is not available to inform the practitioner.

It should be noted that over longer periods of time, the CMAP values can overestimate the number of motor axons. The is because of reinnervation by collateral sprouting that causes each axon to innervate more muscle fibers, and therefore increase the CMAP.

In demyelinating lesions of the plexus, stimulation distal to the injury site will reveal no changes in CMAP amplitudes. Stimulation proximal to the site will demonstrate reduced amplitude secondary to conduction block; however, proximal stimulation is often not possible in root or trunk injury. Instead a positive prognosis can be inferred from the intact distal CMAP amplitudes.

Sensory nerve action potential amplitude

The evaluation of sensory nerve responses in plexopathy offers important diagnostic information. As in CMAP studies, each sensory nerve study will provide information about a different domain of the brachial plexus[5,8] (**Table 2**).

Sensory studies are also key to distinguishing between preganglionic and postganglionic injury. This is based on the anatomy of sensory nerves, which have cell bodies located in the dorsal root ganglion. In axonal lesions distal to the dorsal root ganglion, Wallerian degeneration causes a decrease in the SNAP amplitude by day 6 and with maximum decrease by day 10.

In root avulsions, the dorsal root ganglion and the peripheral axon are spared, leaving the SNAP response intact. Because the sensory fibers proximal to the dorsal root ganglion are damaged, the patient will lack sensation in the corresponding dermatome. It should be noted that absent or diminished SNAP responses do not rule out root avulsion. This is because there may be sufficient force to also cause injury distal to the DRG.

SNAP amplitudes are sensitive for axonal loss in brachial plexus injury. However, because of this sensitivity, sensory responses tend to overestimate the severity of brachial plexus injury and are frequently absent or greatly reduced when less than 50% of the axons are lost.[5]

Needle electromyography: spontaneous activity

Fibrillation potentials and positive sharp waves appear in muscles that have undergone motor axon loss. In muscles near to the injury site, they occur as early as 10 days and in more distal muscles can take up to 4 weeks.[7] In brachial plexopathy, these potentials are primarily used for localization of the lesion. By studying a range of

Table 2
Sensory nerve conduction studies

Study	Root	Trunk	Division	Cord
LABC	C5, C6	Upper (100%)	Anterior	Lateral (100%)
Radial	C6	Upper (60%), middle (40%)	Posterior	Posterior (100%)
Median thumb	C6	Upper (100%)	Anterior	Lateral (100%)
Median index	C6, C7	Upper (20%), middle (80%)	Anterior	Lateral (100%)
Median long	C7	Upper (10%), middle (70%) Lower (20%)	Anterior	Lateral (80%) Medial (20%)
Ulnar small	C8	Lower (100%)	Anterior	Medial (100%)
MABC	C8, T1	Lower (100%)	Anterior	Medial (100%)

muscles with different root, trunk, division, cord, and terminal nerve domains, it is possible to determine which structures are affected[6,7] (**Table 3**).

The presence or grade of spontaneous activity is likely not a useful prognostic indicator. This stems from the difficulty in using spontaneous activity to quantify the extent of axonal loss. The grading scheme for fibrillation potentials and positive sharp waves is an ordinal scale. Therefore, a grade of 4+ fibrillation potentials likely represents

Table 3
Electromyography domains

Muscle	Root	Trunk	Division	Cord	Peripheral Nerve
Root					
Paraspinal	C5-T1				Dorsal ramus
Rhomboid	C5				Dorsal scapular
Serratus Anterior	C5, C6, C7				Long thoracic
Trunk					
Supraspinaus	C5, C6	Upper			Suprascapular
Infraspinatus	C5, C6	Upper			Suprascapular
Cord					
Pectoralis Major	C5, C6, C7	Upper/middle	Anterior	Lateral	Lateral Pectoral
Pectoralis major/minor	C8, T1	Lower	Anterior	Medial	Medial pectoral
Latissimus dorsi	C6, C7, C8	Upper/middle/lower	Posterior	Posterior	Thoracodorsal
Teres major	C5, C6, C7	Upper/middle	Posterior	Posterior	Lower subscapular
Nerve Branch					
Deltoid	C5, C6	Upper	Posterior	Posterior	Axillary
Biceps brachii	C5, C6	Upper	Anterior	Lateral	Musculocutaneous
Brachioradialis	C5, C6	Upper	Posterior	Posterior	Radial
Triceps	C6, C7, C8	Upper/middle/lower	Posterior	Posterior	Radial
Extensor carpi radialis	C6, C7	Upper/middle	Posterior	Posterior	Radial
Pronator teres	C6, C7	Upper/middle	Anterior	Lateral	Median
Extensor digitorum communis	C7, C8	Middle/lower	Posterior	Posterior	Radial
Extensor indicis proprius	C7, C8	Middle/lower	Posterior	Posterior	Radial
Flexor carpi ulnaris	C8, T1	Lower	Anterior	Medial	Ulnar
Flexor carpi radialis	C6, C7, (C8)	Upper/middle/lower	Anterior	Lateral/medial	Median
Abductor pollicus brevis	C8, T1	Lower	Anterior	Medial	Median
Abductor digiti minimi	C8, T1	Lower	Anterior	Medial	Ulnar
First dorsal interosseous	C8, T1	Lower	Anterior	Medial	Ulnar

more axonal loss than 2+ fibrillation potentials; however, one cannot say that it is twice as much or quantify the amount in a prognostically useful way.[9]

Because brachial plexopathy is frequently associated with polytrauma with injury to the central nervous system and direct injury to muscle, care should be taken to ensure that any spontaneous activity observed is caused by brachial plexus injury.

Needle electromyography: recruitment

In the evaluation of brachial plexopathy, voluntary MUAP recruitment is used to provide an estimate of the degree of axonal preservation and to determine if the nerve remains intact. It is additionally used to assess the suitability of donor nerves for nerve transfer surgery.

The effects on voluntary MUAP recruitment observed on needle EMG in brachial plexopathy are immediate. Because voluntary recruitment can be affected both by axonal loss and by conduction block, some caution should be used in interpretation of the findings. Initial evaluation at 3 to 4 weeks may not be able to fully exclude a contribution from conduction block to reduced recruitment. With time, conduction block resolves, and findings can be attributed to axonal loss.

The degree to which recruitment remains intact is an important prognostic indicator, but its limitations should be acknowledged. Because recruitment is described by a subjective ordinal scale, it does not provide an exact quantitative assessment of the degree of axonal loss.

Injuries with full or near full recruitment are likely to make a good recovery. Patients who demonstrate no recruitment or discrete voluntary recruitment at 3 months have a worse prognosis.

In a retrospective review of outcomes in 18 patients with C5, C6 nerve root or upper trunk injury, with electrodiagnosis at an average of 2.5 months and manual muscle testing follow-up greater than 1 year, the authors observed a statistically significant difference in patients who demonstrated no recruitment versus patients who demonstrated discrete recruitment. In patients with no recruitment, 0 of 23 muscles improved to greater than antigravity strength after 1 year. In patients with discrete recruitment, 2 of the 6 muscles (33%) improved to greater than antigravity strength after 1 year. ($P=.037$) (Impastato DM, et al. Prognostic values of electrodiagnostic studies in traumatic brachial plexus injury. Manuscript pending submission.)

Additional Prognostic Factors

Location of injury

The distance between injury site and target muscle for reinnervation plays an important prognostic role. Denervated muscle fibers remain viable for reinnervation for approximately 12 to 18 months. If reinnervation does not occur within this time period, the muscle fibers undergo fibrofatty degradation and become nonviable.[7] Because axonal advancement occurs at a rate of approximately 1 inch per month, lesions that are greater than 18 inches (equivalent to 18 months of nerve regrowth) from the target muscle have a poor prognosis for spontaneous recovery.

The site of injury within the plexus also provides prognostic information. Isolated injuries of the upper trunk have the best prognosis, while injuries to the cords, upper roots, and lower trunk are not as good. Patients with complete plexus injuries have a very poor prognosis.[10]

Kim and colleagues[11] studied the success of nerve repair in brachial plexus injury. Surgical intervention was most successful in injuries located at the C 5 to 7 levels, the upper and middle trunk, and the lateral and posterior cords. Results were poor for injuries at the C8 and T1 levels, and for lower trunk and medial cord lesions.

Root avulsion

Special consideration should be given to the electrodiagnostic identification of nerve root avulsion, as it has important prognostic and surgical implications. Electrodiagnostic findings in root avulsion fit a classic pattern: acute changes in the paraspinals, absent CMAP responses, and intact SNAP responses. The preservation of the SNAP responses is based on the peripheral location of the sensory nerve cell bodies in the dorsal root ganglion. When a nerve root avulsion is identified, prognosis is very poor and will require surgical management to restore function.

SURGICAL INTERVENTION

Over the past several decades, new surgical options have become available to improve functional outcomes after brachial plexus injury. Currently, available options include neurolysis, nerve repair (primary repair vs use of nerve graft), nerve transfer (proximal vs distal), tendon transfer, free functioning muscle transfer (FFMT), and arthrodesis. Of these, perhaps the most exciting developments have been in distal nerve transfer surgery. Proximal nerve transfer occurs in the brachial plexus/neck/shoulder region, with an obligatory long distance for nerve regeneration. Distal nerve transfer occurs near the target muscle, with a much shorter distance required for nerve regeneration (and therefore faster reinnervation of the target muscle, and faster clinical improvement). This article will concentrate on this area, as it is one in which the electrodiagnostician serves not only a diagnostic and prognostic role, but also a role in the identification of suitable donor nerves, especially in preparation for distal nerve transfer.

Timing of Nerve Transfer Surgery

As noted previously, once muscle is denervated, it gradually becomes less viable for reinnervation. Therefore, the timing of surgical intervention is key to achieving maximal functional outcomes. Unfortunately, the optimal timing of surgery occurs before the full extent of spontaneous recovery is achieved, which means the decision to proceed with surgery must be based on the expected prognosis, recovery trajectory, and clinical presentation. Electrodiagnosis plays a key role in prognostication and determining if surgery should be considered. The goal is to identify patients who will not make a good function recovery without intervention, and exclude those who are expected to have good spontaneous recovery with conservative management.

Indications for immediate intervention include penetrating injuries and vascular injuries. This usually involves exploration of the wound with nerve and/or vascular repair. Although a matter of debate, some surgeons recommend early (<3 months) surgical intervention in severe injury, such as with rupture or avulsion. The most common timing for nerve transfer surgery occurs 3 to 6 months following injury. This allows for sufficient time to determine recovery trajectory and to better assess prognosis. It is possible to conduct surgery past this time window, but with diminishing efficacy. The exact time after injury at which nerve repair is considered nonviable is a matter of some debate, but likely occurs around the 12-month window. This applies only to muscles that have been completely denervated. For muscles that are clinically nonfunctional but remained partially innervated, the window for surgical reconstruction may be longer.

Selection of Donor Nerve for Transfer

Electrodiagnostic evaluation

Once it is determined that the prognosis is poor for spontaneous recovery of a specific function, surgical intervention should be considered. The electrodiagnostician plays an essential role in surgical planning by identifying potential donor nerves and excluding unsuitable donor nerves for transfer.

Electrodiagnostic evaluation of potential nerve donors includes both needle EMG and when possible nerve conduction studies. Needle electromyography should emphasize the assessment of voluntary motor unit recruitment, but also note acute denervation and chronic changes in motor unit morphology. Of these variables, voluntary motor unit recruitment has the most evidence for prediction of donor suitability.

Schreiber and colleagues[12] evaluated the outcomes of nerve transfer surgery based on the preoperative assessment of donor motor recruitment on needle EMG. Motor recruitment was defined as full (complete motor unit activation and full interference pattern), decreased (a large quantity of motor units without a full interference pattern and individual units not identified), discrete (a smaller quantity of motor units firing with individual motor units identified during maximum effort.) and none. Subjects with full or decreased recruitment were considered unaffected and donors with discrete recruitment considered affected. Donors with no recruitment were not used for transfer. It should be noted that most transfers were double fascicular and that subjects receiving affected nerves also received 1 unaffected nerve.

Patients in the unaffected cohort (full or decreased recruitment) showed significantly greater improvements in postoperative motor strength when compared with affected (discrete recruitment) donor nerves. ($P<.01$) In a subanalysis of elbow flexion, a trend was observed toward an increased portion (18 of 21; 86%) of patients with the unaffected EMG gaining M4 elbow strength compared with patients in the affected cohort (3 of 6; 50% $P=.06$). In a subanalysis of shoulder abduction, 8 of 8 (100%) of subjects with unaffected EMG gained M4 deltoid strength compared with 0 of 5 (0%) patients in the affected cohort ($P<.001$). In subjects with 2 unaffected fascicles transferred, all patients attained M4 or greater strength. This was statistically significant compared with transfers using 1 normal and 1 affected nerve.

Of note, in the unaffected group, when comparison was made between subjects with full motor unit recruitment and those with decreased recruitment patterns, no statistical significant difference was observed ($P=.44$). Analysis of fibrillation and positive sharp waves effect on outcomes was not undertaken; however, in the unaffected group nearly 50% had the presence of acute changes, and in the affected group 100% had acute changes, with higher-grade changes in the affected group.

The authors' practice is to first identify normal donor nerves with full recruitment, no acute changes, and normal motor unit morphology. However, the electrodiagnostician will not infrequently encounter more extensive plexus injury, where completely normal nerves are not readily available as donors. In these instances, it is reasonable to consider donor nerves that have full or mildly reduced recruitment even in the presence of acute changes. In cases in which 2 donors are transferred, it is reasonable to use 1 donor nerve that has full or near-full recruitment supplemented with a nerve that has a more markedly reduced recruitment.

Surgical evaluation and selection

In addition to the electrodiagnostic evaluation, there are several clinical factors upon which selection of donor nerves depend. First, as indicated by electrodiagnostic study, a healthy donor nerve is critical. Without viable axons from the donor nerve, no nerve regeneration will occur. Second, the length of the donor nerve and recipient nerve is important. Ideally, both donor and recipient nerve endings are long enough to allow coaptation of nerve endings without tension. When the nerve endings are not long enough, a piece of interpositional nerve graft is required to bridge the 2 ends. This creates 2 coaptation sites: one on each side of the nerve graft. This is suboptimal, because when axons regenerate across a coaptation, some will leak out, or get misdirected. Consequently, the more coaptations there are, the smaller the number of regenerating axons that will eventually reach the desired target. Thirdly, nerve synergy is considered. Synergistic nerves are a particular group of nerves that are routinely activated together (eg, wrist extensors and finger flexors are often are activated simultaneously; on the contrary, finger extensors are deactivated when the finger flexors are activated). Synergistic nerve transfers are easier and more intuitive for patients to learn how to use.

Interventions by Functional Deficit

Close communication with surgical providers can identify the exact nerves being considered as donors for transfer, but in general, there are particular sets of donor nerves commonly used for each type of function (**Table 4**).

Shoulder abduction

The restoration of shoulder abduction not only has important functional implications, but can reduce pain associated with shoulder subluxation and glenohumeral instability. Restoring shoulder function is challenging, since the shoulder moves in multiple axes, resulting from coordinated contractions of multiple muscles.

Shoulder function restoration requires reconstruction of 2 nerves: suprascapular and axillary nerves. For suprascapular nerve reconstruction, the spinal accessory nerve is the most commonly used donor nerve. For axillary nerve reconstruction, a triceps branch (medial vs long head) of radial nerve and the medial pectoral nerve are the most common donor nerves. Other reported approaches include phrenic nerve to suprascapular nerve, intercostal nerves to axillary nerve, and thoracodorsal nerve to axillary nerve.[13]

Yang and colleagues[14] reviewed 55 patients who underwent nerve transfers with proximal nerve repair and found that 64% of patients attained and MRC scale score of 3 or higher, and 62% of patients attained in MRC score of 4 or higher. Although not directly comparable, in other studies in patients who received nerve repair alone,

Table 4
Nerve transfer option by target nerve/muscle

	Target		Donor Nerve for Transfer	
	Nerve	**Muscle**	**Nerve**	**Motor Branch**
Shoulder	Suprascapular	Supra/infraspinatus	Spinal accessory	Trapezius
			Phrenic	Diaphragm
	Axillary	Deltoid	Radial	Long/medial head of the triceps
			Medial Pectoral	Pectoralis
			Phrenic	Diaphragm
Elbow	Musculocutaneous	Biceps brachii and brachialis	Medial Pectoral	Pectoral
			Intercostal	Intercostal
			Phrenic	Diaphragm
			Thoracodorsal	Latissimus dorsi
	Musculocutaneous	Biceps brachii	Ulnar	FCU
			Median	FCR/FDS
			Intercostal	Intercostal
	Musculocutaneous	Brachialis	Median	FCR/FDS
	Radial	Triceps	Ulnar	FCU
			Intercostal	Intercostal
Thumb/ finger	Anterior interosseous	FPL, FDS	Musculocutaneous FFMT	Brachialis

only 28% achieved MRC score greater than 3%, and 14% attained a score of four or higher.

Elbow flexion

Restoration of elbow flexion is considered a primary target of surgery. Elbow flexion is accomplished mainly by contraction of 2 muscles; biceps brachii and brachialis. Although biceps brachii flexes the elbow and supinates the forearm, brachialis only flexes the elbow. Both muscles are innervated by branches of the musculocutaneous (MC) nerve. In addition, the MC nerve provides innervation to the skin in the lateral arm/forearm via the lateral antebrachial cutaneous nerve (LABC).

Nerve transfer aimed to restore elbow flexion may target the main MC nerve itself (prior to it branching out to biceps or brachialis), the biceps branch (branches out early from MC, closer to shoulder), or the brachialis branch (branches later from MC, closer to elbow). Although targeting the MC nerve itself may seem like a more anatomic reconstruction, some of the axons from the donor nerve will regenerate into the LABC, which is a sensory nerve and provides no motor function. This is viewed as a waste of donor axons, and therefore, whenever possible, it is preferred to specifically target the biceps branch or the brachialis branch (or both), so all donor axons are directed to reinnervate the desired muscle. If both elbow flexion and forearm supination are desired, then the biceps branch would be preferentially targeted.

To reconstruct the biceps branch, the most commonly used donor is the flexor carpi ulnaris (FCU) fascicle of the ulnar nerve (Oberlin procedure).[15] To reconstruct both the biceps branch and the brachialis branch, FCU fascicle of the ulnar nerve and flexor carpi radialis (FCR) fascicle of the median nerve are used as donor nerves (double fascicular transfer).[16] To reconstruct the MC nerve, intercostal nerves and medial pectoral nerve are commonly used donors.[14]

In 1 systematic review, 91% of patients achieved an MRC scale score of 3, and 71% achieved a score of at least 4 after nerve transfer.[14] In other studies in patients receiving nerve repair alone, 63% of patients regained M3 or higher, and 46% gained M4 or higher. Other available approaches include intercostal nerves transfer to musculocutaneous nerve, thoracodorsal to musculocutaneous nerve,[13] and phrenic nerve to musculocutaneous.[17]

Elbow extension

Elbow extension may be restored by reinnervating the triceps branches of the radial nerve. Reported donor nerves include FCU fascicle of ulnar nerve and intercostal nerves.[18]

Thumb/finger flexion

Thumb flexion may be restored by reinnervating the anterior interosseous nerve (AIN). The brachialis branch of the MC nerve has been used as a donor nerve (brachialis to AIN transfer).[19] When finger flexion is lost because of brachial plexus injury, nerve transfer options are limited, mainly because of the long distance required for nerve regeneration. Often when the regenerating axons reach the finger flexor muscles, the muscles have already undergone irreversible atrophy. In this situation, the atrophic nonfunctional muscle can be replaced with healthy muscle harvested from other parts of the body and transferred using microsurgical technique, also known as free-functioning muscle transfer (FFMT).[20]

Complete brachial plexus injury

Patients with complete brachial plexus injury (C5 – T1) have poor prognosis, and the available options for nerve transfer are often limited. A frequently used approach is to attempt to restore some proximal muscle function aimed at shoulder stability and potentially elbow flexion. Options for transfer in these instances include spinal accessory to suprascapular and intercostals to axillary. More aggressive approaches include use of phrenic nerve,[17] contralateral C7,[21] arthrodesis, and FFMT.[20] In general, hand function cannot be restored because of the limited number of donor nerves for transfer and the distance to the target muscle.

SUMMARY

Brachial plexus injury can severely impact function and quality of life. The management of these injuries is complex, requiring a multidisciplinary team and carefully timed diagnostics and interventions. Electrodiagnostic assessment utilizes detailed knowledge of anatomy and careful application of motor and sensory nerve conduction studies and needle EMG to establish the structures injured and provide prognostic information. Nerve transfer has become a mainstay of surgical intervention to improve the functional outcomes of patients with brachial plexus injury, but this must be carried out within a 3- to 6-month window to achieve optimal outcomes. Electrodiagnosis plays a pivotal role in identifying viable nerve transfer donors through the assessment of voluntary motor unit recruitment.

REFERENCES

1. Gray B. Quality of life following traumatic brachial plexus injury: a questionnaire study. Int J Orthop Trauma Nurs 2016;22:29–35.
2. Midha R. Epidemiology of brachial plexus injuries in a multitrauma population. Neurosurgery 1997;40:1182–8 [discussion: 1188–9].
3. Rhee PC, Pirola E, Hebert-Blouin MN, et al. Concomitant traumatic spinal cord and brachial plexus injuries in adult patients. J Bone Joint Surg Am 2011;93: 2271–7.
4. Emamhadi M, Chabok SY, Samini F, et al. Anatomical variations of brachial plexus in adult cadavers; a descriptive study. Arch Bone Jt Surg 2016;4:253–8.
5. Ferrante MA. Electrodiagnostic assessment of the brachial plexus. Neurol Clin 2012;30:551–80.
6. Ferrante MA. Brachial plexopathies: classification, causes, and consequences. Muscle Nerve 2004;30:547–68.
7. Dumitru D, Amato AA, Zwarts MJ. Electrodiagnostic medicine. 2nd edition. Philadelphia: Hanley & Belfus; 2002.
8. Ferrante MA, Wilbourn AJ. The utility of various sensory nerve conduction responses in assessing brachial plexopathies. Muscle Nerve 1995;18:879–89.
9. Robinson LR. How electrodiagnosis predicts clinical outcome of focal peripheral nerve lesions. Muscle Nerve 2015;52:321–33.
10. Rorabeck CH, Harris WR. Factors affecting the prognosis of brachial plexus injuries. J Bone Joint Surg Br 1981;63-B:404–7.
11. Kim DH, Cho YJ, Tiel RL, et al. Outcomes of surgery in 1019 brachial plexus lesions treated at Louisiana State University Health Sciences Center. J Neurosurg 2003;98:1005–16.
12. Schreiber JJ, Feinberg JH, Byun DJ, et al. Preoperative donor nerve electromyography as a predictor of nerve transfer outcomes. J Hand Surg Am 2014;39: 42–9.
13. Samardzic MM, Grujicic DM, Rasulic LG, et al. The use of thoracodorsal nerve transfer in restoration of irreparable C5 and C6 spinal nerve lesions. Br J Plast Surg 2005;58:541–6.

14. Yang LJ, Chang KW, Chung KC. A systematic review of nerve transfer and nerve repair for the treatment of adult upper brachial plexus injury. Neurosurgery 2012; 71:417–29 [discussion: 429].
15. Oberlin C, Beal D, Leechavengvongs S, et al. Nerve transfer to biceps muscle using a part of ulnar nerve for C5-C6 avulsion of the brachial plexus: anatomical study and report of four cases. J Hand Surg Am 1994;19:232–7.
16. Mackinnon SE, Novak CB, Myckatyn TM, et al. Results of reinnervation of the biceps and brachialis muscles with a double fascicular transfer for elbow flexion. J Hand Surg Am 2005;30:978–85.
17. Liu Y, Xu XC, Zou Y, et al. Phrenic nerve transfer to the musculocutaneous nerve for the repair of brachial plexus injury: electrophysiological characteristics. Neural Regen Res 2015;10:328–33.
18. Gao K, Lao J, Zhao X, et al. Outcome after transfer of intercostal nerves to the nerve of triceps long head in 25 adult patients with total brachial plexus root avulsion injury. J Neurosurg 2013;118:606–10.
19. Ray WZ, Yarbrough CK, Yee A, et al. Clinical outcomes following brachialis to anterior interosseous nerve transfers. J Neurosurg 2012;117:604–9.
20. Maldonado AA, Kircher MF, Spinner RJ, et al. Free functioning gracilis muscle transfer versus intercostal nerve transfer to musculocutaneous nerve for restoration of elbow flexion after traumatic adult brachial pan-plexus injury. Plast Reconstr Surg 2016;138:483e–8e.
21. Mathews AL, Yang G, Chang KW, et al. A systematic review of outcomes of contralateral C-7 transfer for the treatment of traumatic brachial plexus injury: an international comparison. J Neurosurg 2017;126:922–32.

Minimizing Risk of Cancer Therapeutics

Megan Clark, MD

KEYWORDS

- Chemotherapy-induced peripheral neuropathy • Platinum-based toxicity
- Taxane-based toxicity • Radiation fibrosis • Radiation fibrosis syndrome

KEY POINTS

- Chemotherapy-induced peripheral neuropathy (CIPN) is typically a dose-dependent peripheral neuropathy presenting in a "glove and stocking" distribution.
- Typical agents leading to CIPN include use of platinum-based, vinca alkaloid, taxane, proteasome inhibitor, antimicrotubule, and antiangiogenesis drugs.
- Use of ionizing radiation in cancer treatment can lead to radiation fibrosis of tissues involved in the treatment field.
- Radiation fibrosis syndrome (RFS) is the clinical presentation of the resultant damage from progressive fibrotic and sclerotic changes seen in some combination of structures involved.
- Although there are currently no preventive or curative measures for either CIPN or RFS, early diagnosis and treatment can reduce interference with oncologic management and improve patient symptoms and quality of life.

CHEMOTHERAPY-INDUCED PERIPHERAL NEUROPATHY

Chemotherapy-induced peripheral neuropathy (CIPN) is a dose-dependent neuropathy typically presenting in a "glove and stocking" distribution. Affecting 30% to 70% of patients who undergo certain chemotherapeutic treatment,[1] this length-dependent neuropathy typically presents as a sensory peripheral neuropathy, but can also cause motor and autonomic neuropathies. Symptoms usually start after several rounds of the offending chemotherapeutic agent, but they can also have an acute onset or progress even after the discontinuation of treatment.

The pathophysiology leading to CIPN varies slightly between chemotherapy therapeutic agents, but predisposing regimens include the use of platinum-based

Disclosure Statement: No relationship with a commercial company that has a direct financial interest in subject matter or materials discussed in this article or with a company making a competing product.
Oncology Rehabilitation, University of Kansas, Comprehensive Spine Center, 4000 Cambridge Street, Kansas City, KS 66160, USA
E-mail address: Meca8f@gmail.com

Phys Med Rehabil Clin N Am 29 (2018) 701–719
https://doi.org/10.1016/j.pmr.2018.06.006
pmr.theclinics.com
1047-9651/18/© 2018 Elsevier Inc. All rights reserved.

antineoplastic, vinca alkaloid, taxane, proteasome inhibitor, antimicrotubule, and anti-angiogenesis drugs.

At this time, no protective agents used before or during chemotherapy have been found to be effective, but treatment regimens have been used to ameliorate the side effects and symptomatic neuropathy that subsequently develops. Treatment includes a variety of over-the-counter, topical, prescription, and therapeutic options. Even with current treatment options, significant and debilitating neuropathic side effects can require modification of chemotherapeutic treatment regimens and even interruption of the regimen altogether. Continued efforts are undergoing in research and development for protective and symptomatic relief, not only for patient comfort and quality of life,[2,3] but to limit the alteration or cessation of chemotherapeutic regimens because of side effects, such as CIPN.

Chemotherapy-Induced Peripheral Neuropathy Clinical Presentation

Chemotherapy-induced neuropathy is a common side effect of many antineoplastic drug regimens, leading to a length-dependent sensory, motor, and/or autonomic neuropathy. The identification of at-risk patients can be difficult, but identifiable predisposing factors include prior therapy with neurotoxic agents, diabetes mellitus, folate/vitamin B12 deficiencies, African race, and older age.[4,5] Some predisposing causes for peripheral neuropathy can be seen in **Fig. 1**. These variables can impact not only the presence of peripheral neuropathy before treatment, but it can also predispose a patient to develop symptoms early in their treatment course. In these cases, patients should be educated about the risks for neuropathic side effects and monitored closely for development of symptoms. In some situations, as in a patient with neuropathy at presentation, alternative regimens could be considered with agents known to have a lower risk of neurotoxicity.

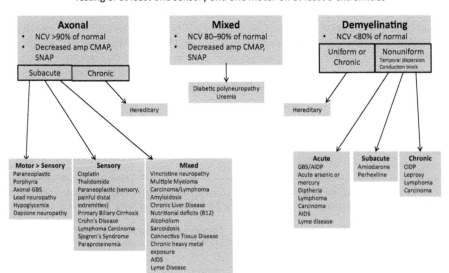

Fig. 1. Peripheral neuropathy diagnostic findings and etiology. AIDP, acute inflammatory demyelinating polyneuropathy; GBS, Guillain-Barré syndrome.

Variability in clinical presentation can be seen among chemotherapeutic agents used, but symptoms typically manifest as a sensory complaint. These symptoms develop first in the feet and hands as a paresthesia or dysesthesia with descriptions of numbness, tingling, stabbing, burning, shooting, tight, or electric shocklike pain. Occasionally, a thermal allodynia and hyperalgesia can occur and can be induced with warm or cool temperatures. Sensory symptoms can be progressive, leading to impaired vibratory sensation and loss of proprioception, leading to disabling ambulatory difficulties. Worsening neuropathic toxicity can lead to a perceived sense of "clumsiness" and subsequent difficulties with upper extremity dexterity, balance, and gait.

Motor neuropathy, although less common than sensory symptoms, can include distal weakness and impaired fine movements. This additionally can lead to disabling symptoms and functional disruption. Vinca alkaloids can lead to distal weakness, including foot drop.

Autonomic symptoms are even less common, but can be present and lead to orthostatic hypotension, constipation, and altered sexual or urinary function.[6] Changes in autonomic functions can be seen in use of vinca alkaloids, taxanes, and platinum compounds.

Typically, the onset of CIPN is dose dependent, but acute neuropathy can be seen in regimens including platinum-based medications and taxanes, specifically oxaliplatin and paclitaxel.[7] A transient neuropathy with dysesthesias and paresthesias of the hands, feet, and perioral region can occur within hours of infusion with use of oxaliplatin. Although this phenomenon has been reported in nearly 90% of patients,[8] it generally resolves between treatment cycles.[9]

Symptoms also can begin or worsen after completion of chemotherapeutic agents. This progressive worsening is described as a "coasting" phenomenon, which can be a persistent and progressive worsening of symptoms over time. Symptoms can progress for 2 to 6 months after the cessation of chemotherapy, which is more often seen with platinum-based treatment and vinca alkaloids to a lesser degree. A cross-sectional study of patients with testicular cancer reevaluated 23 to 33 years after finishing treatment showed that CIPN remains detectable in up to 20% of patients, with 10% of patients being symptomatic.[10] Similar results were found in another study that evaluated cisplatin-treated patients after a median follow-up of 15 years: 38% and 28% of patients had asymptomatic and symptomatic neuropathy, respectively, with "disabling" symptoms in 6%.[11]

Chemotherapy-Induced Peripheral Neuropathy Pathophysiology

There is some variation in the mechanism of action leading to peripheral neuropathy among pharmacologic agents used, but with each regimen the pathophysiology likely is caused by multiple factors. The chemotherapeutic classes commonly implicated in the development of neuropathy include platinum-based antineoplastics, vinca alkaloids, taxanes, proteasome inhibitors, and antimicrotubule and antiangiogenesis agents. These chemotherapeutics, as seen in **Fig. 2**, impact multiple locations including the DNA, mitochondria, and axon transport. Most commonly, microtubule impairment leads to a disruption of the axonal transport and Wallerian degeneration of the nerve. The resultant axonal loss is a typical finding in patients with CIPN.

Chemotherapeutic agents also lead to changes in the excitability of the peripheral nerve. Altered expression and function of ion channels, including voltage-gated sodium, voltage-gated potassium, and transient receptor potential channels, also can contribute to the development of sensory peripheral neuropathy. Altered voltage-gated sodium channels can lead to a significant increase in the duration of the relative

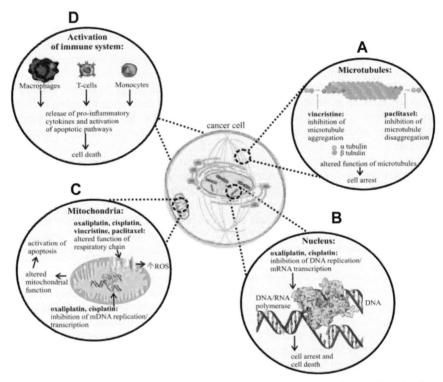

Fig. 2. Chemotherapeutic pathophysiology. ROS, reactive oxygen species mDNA, mitochondrial deoxyribonucleic acid; mRNA, messenger RNA. (*From* Starobova H, Vetter I. Pathophysiology of chemotherapy-induced peripheral neuropathy. Front Mol Neurosci 2017;10:174; with permission.)

refractory period. In mouse studies, oxaliplatin can lead to an increase in current, inhibition of maximal amplitude, and emergence of enhance resurgent and persistent current amplitudes in peripheral axons as well as dorsal root ganglion neurons.[12,13] Decreased expression of potassium channels, particularly seen after oxaliplatin and paclitaxel treatments in rodent models, can further exacerbate altered neuronal excitability.[14,15] Multiple transient receptor potential channels have been studies with regard to their effect on thermosensitive and mechanosensitive pathways.[16–18] There is question currently about the contributions of these individual channel subtypes in CIPN, but the additive disruption of function could act as an adjunct to the disability seen in patients undergoing this treatment.

Chemotherapy-induced peripheral neuropathy pathophysiology: platinum-based chemotherapeutic agents

Platinum-based chemotherapy therapeutic agents, particularly cisplatin and oxaliplatin, frequently are implicated in the development of a distal dose-dependent symmetric sensory CIPN. They are commonly used in the treatment of solid tumors; cisplatin and carboplatin in lung, breast, and ovarian cancers and oxaliplatin as a part of first-line regimens including the FOLFOX (oxaliplatin with fluorouracil and folinic acid) for colorectal cancer therapy. The mechanism of action for platinum-based treatments is to impair tumor cell proliferation. This is done through the interference of cell division and transcription of messenger ribonucleic acid (mRNA) and the inhibition of DNA transcription leading to cell death. The DNA damage and induced apoptosis of the dorsal root ganglion (DRG) neurons is typically thought to be the primary cause of the secondary neurologic symptoms that develop. However, the DRG injury is not thought to be the only mechanism producing drug-specific side effects. Additional activation of the immune system has also been observed, leading to immunogenic cell death. Reactive oxygen species production outside of the cell can result in altered mitochondrial function. Although cisplatin and oxaliplatin can both lead to CIPN, clinically they can present very differently. One explanation for the difference in side effects includes the metabolism of oxaliplatin compared with cisplatin. Oxaliplatin rapidly transforms into reactive dichloro 1,2-diaminocyclohexyl-platinum complex and oxalate. Oxalate is thought to induce dysfunction of the nodal axonal voltage-gated sodium channels.[19] Through this process, the oxalate metabolite has been considered for leading to cold-induced neuropathy seen after treatment with oxaliplatin, but this is not consistently shown.[20] Cisplatin has a variety of dose-limiting side effects, including ototoxicity, nephrotoxicity, myelotoxicity, and neuropathy, which is often one of the most dose-limiting side effects seen with use. Many patients can experience residual neuropathic pain even after improvement in their neuropathy through the "coasting" phenomenon.

Chemotherapy-induced peripheral neuropathy pathophysiology: vinca alkaloid chemotherapeutic agents

Vincristine is a vital component of several chemotherapeutic regimens for adults and children, including CHOP (cyclophosphamide, vincristine, doxorubicin and prednisone), MOPP (mustargen, oncovin [vincristine], procarbazine, prednisone), COPP (cyclophosphamide, vincristine, procarbazine, and prednisone), and BEACOPP (bleomycin, etoposide, doxorubicin, cyclophosphamide, vincristine, procarbazine, and prednisone), which are used for the treatment of numerous cancers, including acute lymphocytic leukemia, acute myeloid leukemia, Hodgkin disease, neuroblastoma, and small-cell lung cancer. It additionally can be used as an immunosuppressant in nonmalignant diseases, such as thrombotic thrombocytopenic purpura or chronic idiopathic thrombocytic purpura. Vinca alkaloids impair the dynamics of microtubules, which are cytoskeletal proteins involved in multiple cell functions. Microtubules are important in the regulation of cell shape, mitosis, chromosome segregation, cell division, and cellular transport. Disruption of the microtubule aggregation can lead to mitotic arrest,[21] and a loss of axonal microtubules causes axonopathy through axonal transport impairment.[22] Variable affinity for tubulin among the vinca alkaloid compounds has been attributed to the difference in clinical neurotoxicity.[23] Sensory symptoms are seen early in treatment, but vincristine toxicity also can cause distal motor weakness, neuropathic pain, and autonomic dysfunction.[24]

Chemotherapy-induced peripheral neuropathy pathophysiology: taxane chemotherapeutic agents

Paclitaxel and docetaxel are typically used in treatments for solid tumors, including breast, prostate, lung, pancreatic, and gynecologic diagnoses. Both of these drugs act in the disruption of microtubules by inhibiting the disassembly of tubulin from the microtubule polymer. This interruption of the microtubule formation and function can lead to axonopathy. Although both have similar mechanisms of action, subtle difference in their pharmacology can lead to distinct clinical effects. Neither compound crosses the blood-brain barrier; however, it has been noted that paclitaxel accumulates in the DRG neurons to a higher degree than docetaxel[25] and is slightly more neurotoxic. Other taxanes, such as cablitaxel, have a reduced frequency of CIPN, but can present with other neurotoxic side effects including optic neuropathy.

Chemotherapy-induced peripheral neuropathy pathophysiology: proteasome inhibitor chemotherapeutic agents

Proteasome inhibitors inhibit the 26S proteasome, suppress secretion of cytokines in the bone marrow, and enhance oxidative stress. Neuropathy seen with use of these drugs is predominantly sensory, with involvement of the small fibers leading to neuropathic pain. Autonomic changes, including postural hypotension, are possible. Bortezomib is a derivative of boronic acid and used as treatment in mantle cell lymphoma and occasionally in combination with thalidomide in treatment of multiple myeloma. CIPN is seen in approximately 50% of the patients receiving treatment with bortezomib,[26] with a dose-dependent relationship to severity of symptoms observed. However, the mechanism of action of bortezomib, inhibition of the 26S proteasome, has not been linked to the pathogenesis of CIPN.[2] It is thought that it works on both the DRG and peripheral nerves to interfere with transcription, nuclear processing, and cytoplasmic translation of mRNA.[27] This could lead to damage of large finger and C-fibers with abnormal vesicular inclusion bodies in unmyelinated axons.[28] Carfilzomib is a new proteasome inhibitor with reportedly fewer neurotoxic adverse effects.[29]

Chemotherapy-induced peripheral neuropathy pathophysiology: antimicrotubule chemotherapeutic agents

Working similarly to taxanes, epothilones also enhance tubulin polymerization and disruption axonal transport. Fewer patients have been studied with regard to sensory side effects in the use of epothilones. Sensory neuropathy has been variable, with 6% to 71% of patients with clinically significant symptoms.[30] Ixabepilone is an epothilone analog that can be used alone or in conjunction with capecitabine in the treatment of locally advanced or metastatic breast cancer. Eribulin is distinct in its effect as a microtubule dynamics inhibitor from epothilones and taxanes. It is used in treatment of patients with locally advanced or metastatic breast cancer and in patients with liposarcoma. Initial trials are hopeful in the reduced side-effect profile of eribulin with a relatively low incidence and severity of neuropathy.[31]

Chemotherapy-induced peripheral neuropathy pathophysiology: antiangiogenesis chemotherapeutic agents

The common chemotherapeutic agents with antiangiogenesis mechanisms include thalidomide and lenalidomide. Thalidomide is used in the treatment of multiple myeloma both singularly and in combination. The exact mechanisms for the neurotoxic effects seen with the use of thalidomide are unknown, but can be irreversible and unrelated to the dose.[32] Lenalidomide is typically used after treatment with bortezomib in recurrent mantle cell lymphoma, in multiple myeloma in combination with dexamethasone, or as a maintenance therapy following autologous stem cell transplantation. Both thalidomide and lenalidomide can cause a sensory neuropathy, but patients also can present with perioral neuropathic symptoms.

Chemotherapy-Induced Peripheral Neuropathy Diagnosis

Although the incidence of CIPN can be variable depending on drug regimen use, synergistic neurotoxicity from concurrent or prior chemotherapeutics, cumulative dose, and patient comorbidities, the reported prevalence can reach nearly 100% for some agents.[1] Many of the studies that have reported on the symptoms of CIPN have relied on grading scales, patient-reported outcomes, questionnaires, and to a lesser degree objective assessments such as quantitative sensory testing or nerve conduction studies.[33] There are a multitude of scenarios that might lead a provider to consider additional tests and interventions, not only when a patient presents with neurotoxicity symptoms but even before their treatment (**Table 1**).

Table 1
Indications for additional testing before chemotherapy treatment

History and Physical Examination Findings	Example	Diagnostic Options	Treatment
Neck or low back pain	Patient with history of cervical or lumbar pain with pain, numbness, or tingling in extremities	Evaluation for spinal stenosis including consideration for additional imaging and NCS/EMG	Treatment of underlying cause as indicated to limit delay in treatment or worsening of symptoms.
Numbness or tingling in bilateral hands or feet	History of diabetes or metabolic syndrome History of gastric bypass History of heavy alcohol use	NCS/EMG can identify the presence and severity of a baseline neuropathy	Chemotherapeutic regimens can be augmented to limit the neurotoxicity as needed.
Numbness or tingling in unilateral or bilateral fingers/hands	Patient with unilateral or bilateral symptoms involving upper extremity	NCS/EMG for evaluation of mononeuropathy	Carpal tunnel treatment (behavioral adjustment, resting wrist splint, interventional management).
High risk for disability	Elderly, African American, lower socioeconomic status	Identification of patient-specific risk factors	Multidisciplinary treatment and education to limit disability and improve compliance.
Difficulty with balance or mobility	Elderly patient History of dizziness or vertigo History of frequent falls or limited mobility	Timed Up and Go testing Underlying vestibular involvement	Physical therapy for fall prevention training, strengthening, balance directed exercises before treatment. Consider vestibular therapy as indicated.
Limited social or home support	Patient who lives alone No close family or friends available for assistance	Identification of patient-specific risk factors	Develop patient-centered support with information on available services and support groups in the area.

Abbreviations: EMG, electromyography; NCS, nerve conduction study.

Questionnaires have been created to capture the patient self-report of symptoms and functional limitations. One such questionnaire, the European Organization for Research and Treatment of Cancer Quality of Life Questionnaire-CIPN 20-item scale (QLQ-CIPN20), is a 20-item survey used to identify the subjective symptoms by patients by quantifying the symptoms and impairments of sensory, motor, and autonomic neuropathy.[34] This is commonly used in large oncology clinical trials to help try to standardize the symptoms and impact on patients. Grading scales also are used, including the National Cancer Institute Common Toxicity Criteria, Eastern Cooperative Oncology Group criteria,[35] and World Health Organization criteria.[36] Although the use of such forms can be helpful in categorizing subjective complaints, they can be limited when used alone, given the inherent variability of these types of evaluations.[37] Early clinical suspicion is beneficial for the identification of neurotoxic side effects, but may be more beneficial when used in conjunction with objective measures for accurate diagnosis and treatment.

Neurophysiological tests can be used as an objective measure in CIPN. Nerve conduction velocity (NCV) measurements of sensory nerve action potential (SNAP), compound muscle action potential (CMAP), and needle electromyography (EMG) are standard evaluations used.[38] Peripheral neuropathy can be a difficult picture to sort out with multiple etiologies, as described earlier, but these variable causes can have subtle differences in nerve conduction study (NCS)/EMG findings, as seen in **Fig. 1**. Chemotherapy primarily leads to peripheral neuropathy by inducing alteration of microtubule function, which impairs the anterograde and retrograde axonal transport and leads to Wallerian degeneration of the peripheral nerves. Axonal loss is a typical finding in patients with CIPN, and is seen as a reduced amplitude of SNAP and CMAP with mildly reduced conduction velocities.[33,39]

The variable pathophysiology of chemotherapeutic regimens can present with a range of impairments including loss of large myelinated, small unmyelinated, and intraepidermal nerve cells. Although typical changes seen demonstrate axon degeneration following the administration of chemotherapeutic agents, there is likely an additional contribution of supplementary mechanisms that lead to the variation in presenting symptoms (**Table 2**). Although the direct toxic effects on the axons will intuitively lead to neuropathic side effects, indirect effects of gene expression likely also contribute to CIPN. Indirect effects through gene expression and alterations to cellular DNA suggest additional mechanisms that can contribute to the direct damage of peripheral nerves. Electrophysiologic tests evaluate the integrity of large myelinated populations, and can be useful in evaluation of regimens that cause either demyelination or degeneration of large myelinated axons, but are insensitive to degeneration of unmyelinated axons in early stages of neuropathy. Loss of myelin and changes to axonal cytoskeleton can contribute to the sensory and motor symptoms, but this contribution from demyelination is not entirely clear. When small sensory fibers are involved in the pathogenesis, there can be poor correlation between changes in NCV and clinical findings.

Platinum-based

Platinum compounds can lead to distal, symmetric, and sensorimotor polyneuropathy. With damage more commonly seen to the DRG, findings can include sensory neuronopathy, including sensory ataxia and a reduction or loss of SNAP seen to a greater degree in the upper extremities compared with the lower extremities.[40] With higher cisplatin dosage, reduced sensory nerve action potentials and loss of large myelinated fibers also can be seen.[41] Cisplatin-induced CIPN typically affects the periphery and can include a mix of sensory and motor symptoms. Cisplatin led to diminished action potential amplitude and reduced NCV in studies of the sciatic nerve in mice.[42] Motor NCV measures in patients with decreased fiber irritation sensitivity, loss of ankle jerk, and paresthesia showed loss of sural nerve response.[43] Oxaliplatin leads to a moderate sensory-motor axonal degeneration with loss of intraepidermal nerve fibers.[44]

Vinca alkaloid

Degeneration of distal sensory axons, secondary demyelination, and nerve fiber loss has also been reported in vincristine-induced neuropathy.[42,45] Electrophysiological testing in patients with CIPN after treatment with a vinca alkaloid will demonstrate reduced or absent sural nerve potentials.

Table 2
Chemotherapeutic agent common clinical and electrodiagnostic findings

Family	Common Medications Used (Generic)	Mechanism of Peripheral Neurotoxicity	Symptoms	Electrodiagnostic Findings	Additional Findings
Platinum-based agents	Cisplatin (Platinol) Oxaliplatin (Eloxatin)	Interference of cell division and transcription of mRNA Impaired axonal transport	Sensory neuropathy Cold-induced neuropathy (oxaliplatin) Ototoxicity, nephrotoxicity, myelotoxicity (cisplatin)	Axonal sensory and motor polyneuropathy Decreased or absent SNAP	"Coasting" phenomenon common May have severe and irreversible damage with first cycle
Taxanes	Paclitaxel (Taxol) Docetaxel (Taxotere)	Disruption of microtubules with toxic effects to the neuronal cell body and/ or axon	Acute myalgia Dose-dependent sensory neuropathy Sensorimotor (rare)	Axonal sensory and motor polyneuropathy Decreased sural SNAP amplitude Decreased tibial CMAP amplitude Variable asymmetry	Paclitaxel accumulates in the DRG to a higher degree
Vinca alkaloids	Vincristine (Oncovin) Vinorelbine (Navelbine) Vinblastine (Velban)	Impaired microtubule aggregation and axonal transport	Sensory neuropathy Distal motor weakness Occasional cranial nerve and/or autonomic dysfunction	Distal sensory axonal loss Secondary demyelination	Acute taste impairment Lower incidence of neuropathy with Vinblastine
Proteasome inhibitors	Bortezomib (Velcade) Carfilzomib (Kyprolis)	Suppressed cytokine secretion. Unknown mechanism for peripheral neurotoxicity	Sensory neuropathy Small fiber neuropathy	Axonal loss	Reduced incidence with subcutaneous dosing
Microtubule inhibitors	Ixabepilone (Ixempra) Eribulin (Halaven)	Enhanced tubulin polymerization	Sensory neuropathy Sensorimotor (rare)	Demyelinating Can present with myokymia (eribulin)	Rare autonomic dysfunction seen
Antiangiogenesis	Thalidomide (Thalomid) Lenalidomide (Revlimid)	Unknown mechanism for peripheral neurotoxicity	Sensory neuropathy Small fiber neuropathy	Axonal neuropathy Reduced SNAP	Perioral neuropathic symptoms

Abbreviations: CMAP, compound muscle action potential; DRG, dorsal root ganglion; mRNA, messenger RNA; SNAP, sensory nerve action potential.

Taxanes

Taxanes typically produce an axonal sensory-motor polyneuropathy secondary to damage to the axonal microtubule system. In a study by Chen and colleagues,[46] electrodiagnostic evaluation of 55 women with clinical symptoms of polyneuropathy were evaluated with NCS, including CMAP in median, ulnar, peroneal, and tibial nerves; SNAP in median, ulnar, radial, and sural nerves; and needle EMG. In this study, 67% of patients were diagnosed with a mild to severe sensory-motor polyneuropathy with severity that correlated with cumulative dose received. Additionally, examiners found frequent asymmetry, high sural and radial sensory amplitude ratio in patients with mild polyneuropathy, and slow conduction velocity seen only at the common entrapment sites, such as the carpal tunnel.

Chemotherapy-Induced Peripheral Neuropathy Prevention and Treatment

Although the current pathophysiology and mechanism that lead to neuronal dysfunction and symptomatic neuropathy is unclear in the development of CIPN, multiple prevention and treatment options have been used in managing the development of the symptoms. At this time, there has not been a consistent intervention that has proven effective in the prevention of neuropathic symptoms. Preventive drugs can potentially counteract cancer therapy. This has been the problem with several previously used preventive therapies. Several drugs have been used, such as vitamins B and E, glutathione, alpha lipoic acid, acetylcysteine, amifostine, calcium and magnesium, diethyldithiocarbamate, dithiocarbamate, Org 2766, oxcarbazepine,[47] and erythropoietin.[48] For platinum drugs, a Cochrane review states that chemoprotective agents do not seem to prevent CIPN.[49] Continued efforts are being made to address this, and as our understanding of the dominant mechanisms contributing to these symptoms progresses, future elimination of these significant side effects continues to be attempted.

Currently, treatment strategies for CIPN include modification of the chemotherapy regimen, alteration of dosage, and adjustment of treatment cycles, timing, dosage form, and duration. Symptomatic management is also attempted and can use a variety of treatments, including supplements, topical medications, prescription medications, and therapeutic modalities. Although none of the current treatment options reverses the neuropathy that is present, they can work to ameliorate the symptoms. Much of the current treatment regimens use neuromodulating medications, including anticonvulsants and antidepressants, which have proven efficacy in other forms of neuropathy, such as diabetic peripheral neuropathy. In a study by Smith and colleagues,[50] duloxetine was demonstrated as a beneficial treatment over placebo in the treatment of CIPN. Still, at this time no definitive preventive or symptomatic treatment for CIPN exists, and, if not diagnosed and managed early, neurotoxic side effects can force chemotherapeutic dose reduction, break in treatment, or discontinuation of the agent completely.

RADIATION FIBROSIS

Radiation therapy (XRT) is one of the primary treatments used in curative and palliative management in multiple cancers. Through the use of ionizing radiation, rapidly dividing tumor cells are targeted by direct damage to the cells and indirect ionization leading to free radical formation. Radiation fibrosis (RF) can develop in normal tissue included in the treatment field through the accumulation of abnormal protein and fibrin. Multiple radiation-induced symptoms can be seen with RF, and RF syndrome (RFS) describes "the myriad of clinical manifestations of progressive fibrotic tissue sclerosis resulting from radiation treatment."[51] Neuromuscular chronic and cumulative effects are commonly seen in patients with head and neck cancer (HNC) or Hodgkin lymphoma (HL), but can be seen in other tumor types requiring high doses of radiation through key neurologic structures. This damage can manifest as a "myelo-radiculo-plexo-neuro-myopathy" and involve damage to the spinal cord, nerve roots, plexus, peripheral nerves, and muscles, contributing to a complicated web of presenting symptoms.[52] Diagnosis of this damage requires detailed clinical history taking, including tumor type/location, total radiation dose, radiation dose per fraction, concomitant treatment received, and comorbid medical history. Objective testing also may be beneficial in shifting through possible etiologies to determine the correct diagnosis. Localizing and describing the cause of a patient's neuromuscular symptoms can be aided with use of electrodiagnostic testing as an extension of the clinical history and physical examination. Once identified and properly diagnosed, management of these side effects often requires a multidisciplinary team to address the symptomatic and functional effects seen in the days to years following XRT.

Radiation Fibrosis Clinical Presentation

Onset of symptoms after XRT can be seen in days, weeks, months, and even years following treatment. The systems affected can be variable, with all tissues in the treatment area vulnerable to injury, leading to a variety of presentations (**Table 3**). Acute side effects, such as nausea and fatigue, are typically self-limited and resolve over time. Changes in the skin or radiodermatitis are acute and chronic changes in the integumentary system that can present as pigmentation changes, photosensitivity, telangiectasia, fibrosis, atrophy, and delayed wound healing. Neuromuscular complications can present following damage to any neural or muscular structure within the radiation field, including the spinal cord, nerve roots, cranial, cervical or brachial plexus, peripheral nerve, or muscle. These injuries can present as sensory impairment, neuropathic pain, weakness, gait disturbance, activities of daily living dysfunction, and even autonomic changes in blood pressure, bowel, bladder, and sexual function. Because of the multitude of structures that can be involved, describing as such ("myelo-radiculo-plexo-neuro-myopathy"[53]) through the appropriate history and physical examination can better elucidate the etiology behind the symptoms.

Radiation Fibrosis Pathophysiology

Although the pathophysiology leading to neurotoxic effects is not yet fully understood, it involves an additive and chronic change of the intracellular and extracellular matrix within the radiation treatment field. Acute trauma is noted in response to radiotherapy, but repetitive injuries throughout the treatment course can lead to the progressive and characteristic changes seen in these patients.[54] The local damage leads to an initial microvascular injury, which progresses through an evolution with a prefibrotic, fibrotic, and late fibro-atrophic phase.[55] In radiation, both proinflammatory and anti-inflammatory effects are seen,[56] which are dose and schedule dependent. As in typical tissue injury, inflammation, with activation of macrophages and fibroblasts, stimulates fibrogenesis and granulation tissue formation. Injury to tissue, particularly endothelial cells, leads to an initial activation of the coagulation system. Impaired thrombin utilization creates an inflammatory environment. It has been thought that ischemic changes lead to chronic hypoxia and predisposed cells to develop RF. More recent beliefs include a change in the microvascularization secondary to proinflammatory effects of thrombin, which induce an intermittent rather than chronic hypoxia.[57] The endothelial damage, proliferation of thrombin, continued fibrin accumulation, and circulating reactive oxygen species could contribute to the progressive fibrosis leading to RF and contributing to the development of RFS.

Table 3
Indications for additional testing before or after radiation

History and Physical Examination Findings	Example	Diagnostic Options	Treatment
Neck atrophy and weakness (neck drop)	Patient has pain involving the neck and even difficulty maintaining a normal upright posture	EMG with myopathic motor units in affected muscles Muscle biopsy can show nemaline rod myopathy (not routinely done)	Physical therapy to work with improved posture and body mechanics with education on the importance of lifelong independent maintenance with home exercise program.
Neck or low back pain	Patient with history of cervical or lumbar pain with pain, numbness, or tingling in extremities	Evaluation for compressive radiculopathy including consideration for additional imaging and NCS/EMG	Treatment of underlying cause as indicated to limit delay in treatment or worsening of symptoms following radiation.
Numbness or tingling in bilateral hands or feet	History of chemotherapy use History of predisposing etiology for peripheral neuropathy	NCS/EMG can identify the presence and severity of a peripheral neuropathy	Neuromodulator medications to help alleviate symptoms. Therapy as indicated for fall prevention training, strengthening, and balance directed exercises.
Weakness and pain in either upper or lower extremities	Patient with radiation involving the brachial and/or lumbosacral plexus	Electrodiagnostic testing can help to distinguish from plexopathy vs radiculopathy (although they can commonly be seen together)	
Numbness or tingling in unilateral or bilateral fingers/hands	Patient with unilateral or bilateral symptoms involving upper extremity May have history of radiation to an extremity (sarcoma or Hodgkin)	NCS/EMG for evaluation of radiculopathy or mononeuropathy	Can precipitate or exacerbate premorbid condition. Carpal tunnel treatment (ergonomic modifications, resting wrist splint, interventional management).
Shoulder pain and dysfunction	Impingement syndrome Rotator cuff tendonitis Adhesive capsulitis	Clinical examination Imaging (if atypical presentation or not responsive to conservative treatment) Electrodiagnostic tests may show plexopathy (upper), radiculopathy (C5 or C6)	Address primary deficiency (rotator cuff weakness, tightness of the pectoral girdle, restoration of normal anatomic alignment) with physical therapy/home exercise program. Anti-inflammatory treatment with medications and/or sub-acromial injections to improve participation with therapy.

Abbreviations: EMG, electromyography; NCS, nerve conduction study.

Current radiation delivery strategies include use of external beam radiation and brachytherapy, which deliver radiation from outside or inside the body respectively. The delivery of radiation continues to evolve with more focused techniques such as intensity-modulated radiotherapy (IMRT) and image-guided radiotherapy (IGRT). IMRT uses multidirectional radiation beams to deliver focused and precise treatment.[58] With improved radiation techniques and the use of targeted 3-dimensional conformal XRT, dosages to nearby tissues are reduced with more focused treatment of the tumor. Attempts to limit the radiation dose to normal tissue have been made in hopes of decreasing secondary side effects, but our current treatments continue to have a risk of neuromuscular injury.[59] Understanding of the dose delivery (including the total dose of delivery and the dose per treatment), radiation field (including type of tissue radiated), time from treatment, and additional treatments received will be critical in the evaluation and diagnosis of secondary effects.[60]

Radiation Fibrosis Diagnosis

Use of electrodiagnostic (EDX) techniques can aid in the diagnosis and extent of radiation-induced toxicity. In the complicated clinical picture that can present with RFS, EDX can help to untangle layered neuromuscular disorders. Testing should be performed with the guidance of a thorough history and physical examination. Improved understanding of the patient's history (primary tumor, treatment, current disease status) and symptoms can help to lead the evaluation. Chemotherapy-induced neuropathy, as described earlier, will present as a low-amplitude SNAP more commonly seen in the lower than upper extremities. This also can be seen in a variety of preexisting medical conditions as described earlier, and a patient's history may be helpful in differentiating cause. Studies should evaluate all levels of the peripheral nervous system through the known radiation field, including nerve roots, plexus, peripheral nerves, and muscles. Additional upper extremity motor and sensory nerves also can be included as needed to help determine level of injury. For example, patients with HNC or HL commonly develop RFS following XRT. Given the areas involved in the field of radiation, radiation-induced brachial plexopathy is frequently seen. Findings of EDX can help to determine location of injury and distinguish between a neoplastic and radiation-induced injury. Neoplastic symptoms that can be confused for or are concomitant with RFS neuropathy are typically painful and preferentially affect the lower trunk (**Table 4**).

NCSs are important in the evaluation of the peripheral nervous system to help distinguish peripheral involvement. To evaluate this completely, bilateral SNAP and CMAP (typically of the ulnar nerve to reduce confounding median mononeuropathy) as well as one lower extremity SNAP and CMAP should be tested in a patient in whom RFS is suspected. This type of diagnostic test can be helpful in determining the presence of upper extremity changes as seen in plexopathy and ganglionopathy (**Fig. 3**).

Table 4 Neoplastic and radiation-induced plexopathy	
Neoplastic	**Radiation-Induced**
Lower trunk (historically)	Myokymia and fasciculation potentials
Acute onset	Delayed onset
Commonly report pain	Pain less common
	Progressive weakness/paresthesia

Note, overlapping findings are not uncommon and may indicate additional investigation (ie, MRI).

Nerve Conduction Study

Bilateral upper (ie, ulnar nerve) and unilateral
lower extremity SNAP and CMAP testing

-Low amplitude or absent UE SNAP
-Preserved or relatively preserved LE SNAP

- Bilateral Plexopathy (seen in HNC and HL cancers)
- Sensory Ganglionopathy (seen following platinum-based
  treatment and paraneoplastic)

Fig. 3. Sensory NCS findings in suspected RFS. LE, lower extremity; UE, upper extremity.

Low-amplitude or absent upper extremity SNAPs, with preserved or relatively preserved lower extremity SNAPs, may suggest bilateral plexopathy. However, this un-
usual pattern also may suggest a sensory ganglionopathy (a non–length-dependent
form of CIPN) from exposure to platinum-based chemotherapy or from a paraneoplastic disorder.[61] Upper plexopathies, affecting the sensory nerves, such as lateral antebrachial cutaneous, are more common than lower plexopathies in patients with HNC
or HL.

EMG testing should include a general screen for each root level in an involved area,
but additional proximal muscle testing can be considered when evaluating for RFS.
EMG testing within the radiation field can be difficult and present with myopathic,
neuropathic, and fibrotic findings as seen in **Fig. 4**. Spontaneous activity, motor unit
remodeling, and reduced recruitment also can be demonstrated with myokymic discharges and fasciculation potentials. Myopathic changes are seen as low-amplitude
CMAPs, short duration, polyphasia, and early recruitment. Neurogenic changes with
large, long-duration, polyphasic motor units with neurogenic recruitment can be present in a variable proportion. EMG testing in fibrotic muscle shows low-amplitude,
short-duration, polyphasic motor unit potential with normal or deceased insertional
activity and rare fibrillation potentials.[62]

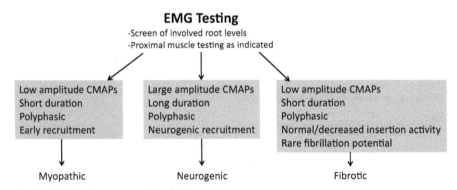

EMG Testing
-Screen of involved root levels
-Proximal muscle testing as indicated

Low amplitude CMAPs	Large amplitude CMAPs	Low amplitude CMAPs
Short duration	Long duration	Short duration
Polyphasic	Polyphasic	Polyphasic
Early recruitment	Neurogenic recruitment	Normal/decreased insertion activity
		Rare fibrillation potential

Myopathic   Neurogenic   Fibrotic

Fig. 4. EMG findings in suspected RFS.

Somatosensory evoked potentials (SEPs) can be used to evaluate transmission from the periphery to the cortex and can be helpful if there is concern for the presence of myelopathy. Particularly in patients with HNC or HL, an SEP from the lower extremities could be used. However, patients with significant peripheral neuropathy cannot reliably isolate deficits to the central nervous system.

Radiation Fibrosis Prevention and Treatment

As briefly described previously, presenting symptoms seen in RFS can be variable. The clinical presentation can be confusing with the multitude of systems affected within a treatment field. Although there is no current treatment to stop the progression of RF, the symptoms of RFS can be ameliorated. These progressive fibrotic changes make early identification and management key to improved function and quality of life.

A team approach with a comprehensive cancer care model of rehabilitation is needed to encompass the multidimensional aspects involved in optimization of function and minimization of symptoms.[63] Physical therapy continues to be a mainstay with stressed importance for lifetime individual maintenance to limit the progressive disability that can be seen with fibrotic changes. Patients have to be empowered with the education of the neuromuscular and musculoskeletal deficits that can develop and work with their therapists to create an individualized exercise and stretching program. Lymphatic therapy also can be important to mitigate RFS symptoms through complex decongestive therapy, including skin care, exercise, manual lymphatic drainage, and compression dressing. Interventional treatment options can be considered in symptomatic treatment for patients with RFS. In cases of myofascial pain, trigger point injections can be helpful to temporarily provide local pain relief. Additional interventional treatment with botulinum toxin injections is used in a variety of instances, including spasticity, spasm, and neuropathic and musculoskeletal pain. This treatment can be beneficial in specific complications of RFS, including trismus, cervical dystonia secondary to radiation, muscle spasms, and focal neuropathic pain disorders.[64]

With appropriate clinical evaluation, physical examination, electrodiagnostic evaluation, and diagnosis, the rehabilitation, management, and treatment can become more focused. This not only aids in focusing the approach based on the primary etiology, but also reduces unnecessary medical and therapeutic management of misdiagnosed symptoms.

REFERENCES

1. Seretny M, Currie GL, Sena ES, et al. Incidence, prevalence, and predictors of chemotherapy-induced peripheral neuropathy: a systematic review and meta-analysis. Pain 2014;155:2461–70.
2. Grisold W, Cavaletti G, Windebank AJ. Peripheral neuropathies from chemotherapeutics and targeted agents: diagnosis, treatment, and prevention. Neuro Oncol 2012;14(Suppl. 4):iv45–54.
3. Jones D, Zhao F, Brell J, et al. Neuropathic symptoms, quality of life, and clinician perception of patient care in medical oncology outpatients with colorectal, breast, lung, and prostate cancer. J Cancer Surviv 2015;9:1–10.
4. Hausheer FH, Schilsky RL, Bain S, et al. Diagnosis, management, and evaluation of chemotherapy-induced peripheral neuropathy. Semin Oncol 2006;33(1):15–49.
5. Schneider BP, Li L, Radovich M, et al. Genome-wide association studies for taxane-induced peripheralneuropathy (TIPN) in ECOG-5103 and ECOG-1199. Clin Cancer Res 2015;21(22):5082–91.

6. Mols F, van de Poll-Franse LV, Vreugdenhil G, et al. Reference data of the European Organization for Research and Treatment of Cancer (EORTC) QLQ-CIPN20 questionnaire in the general Dutch population. Eur J Cancer 2016;69:28–38.

7. Loprinzi CL, Reeves BN, Dakhil SR, et al. Natural history of paclitaxel-associated acute pain syndrome: prospective cohort study NCCTG N08C1. J Clin Oncol 2011;29:1472–8.

8. Argyriou AA, Cavaletti G, Briani C, et al. Clinical pattern and associations of oxaliplatin acute neurotoxicity: a prospective study in 170 patients with colorectal cancer. Cancer 2013;119:438–44.

9. Extra JM, Marty M, Brienza S, et al. Pharmacokinetics and safety profile of oxaliplatin. Semin Oncol 1998;25:13–22.

10. Glendenning JL, Barbachano Y, Norman AR, et al. Long-term neurologic and peripheral vascular toxicity after chemotherapy treatment of testicular cancer. Cancer 2010;116:2322–31.

11. Strumberg D, Brugge S, Korn MW, et al. Evaluation of long-term toxicity in patients after cisplatin-based chemotherapy for non-seminomatous testicular cancer. Ann Oncol 2002;13:229–36.

12. Adelsberger H, Quasthoff S, Grosskreutz J, et al. The chemotherapeutic oxaliplatin alters voltage-gated Na(+) channel kinetics on rat sensory neurons. Eur J Pharmacol 2000;406:25–32.

13. Sittl R, Lampert A, Huth T, et al. Anticancer drug oxaliplatin induces acute cooling-aggravated neuropathy via sodium channel subtype Na(V) 1.6-resurgent and persistent current. Proc Natl Acad Sci U S A 2012;109:6704–9.

14. Descoeur J, Pereira V, Pizzoccaro A, et al. Oxaliplatin-induced cold hypersensitivity is due to remodeling of ion channel expression in nociceptors. EMBO Mol Med 2011;3:266–78.

15. Zhang H, Dougherty PM. Enhanced excitability of primary sensory neurons and altered gene expression of neuronal ion channels in dorsal root ganglion in paclitaxel-induced peripheral neuropathy. Anesthesiology 2014;120:1463–75.

16. Nassini R, Gees M, Harrison S, et al. Oxaliplatin elicits mechanical and cold allodynia in rodents via TRPA1 receptor stimulation. Pain 2011;152:1621–31.

17. Yamamoto K, Chiba N, Chiba T, et al. Transient receptor potential ankyrin 1 that is induced in dorsal root ganglion neurons contributes to acute cold hypersensitivity after oxaliplatin administration. Mol Pain 2015;11:69.

18. Mizoguchi S, Andoh T, Yakura T, et al. Involvement of c-Myc-mediated transient receptor potential melastatin 8 expression in oxaliplatin-induced cold allodynia in mice. Pharmacol Rep 2016;68:645–8.

19. Krishnan AV, Goldstein D, Friedlander M, et al. Oxaliplatin-induced neurotoxicity and the development of neuropathy. Muscle Nerve 2005;32:51–60.

20. Deuis JR, Zimmermann K, Romanovsky AA, et al. An animal model of oxaliplatin-induced cold allodynia reveals a crucial role for Nav1.6 in peripheral pain pathways. Pain 2013;154:1749–57.

21. Gan PP, McCarroll JA, Po'uha Kamath K, et al. Microtubule dynamics, mitotic arrest, and apoptosis: drug-induced differential effects of betaIII-tubulin. Mol Cancer Ther 2010;9:1339–48.

22. Sahenk Z, Brady ST, Mendell JR. Studies on the pathogenesis of vincristine-induced neuropathy. Muscle Nerve 1987;10:80–4.

23. Lobert S, Vulevic B, Correia JJ. Interaction of vinca alkaloids with tubulin: a comparison of vinblastine, vincristine, and vinorelbine. Biochemistry 1996;35:6806–14.

24. Dougherty PM, Cata JP, Curton AW, et al. Dysfunction in multiple primary afferent fiber subtypes revealed by quantitative sensory testing in patients with chronic vincristine-induced pain. J Pain Symptom Manage 2007;33:166–79.

25. Wozniak KM, Vornov JJ, Wu Y, et al. Sustained accumulation of microtubule-binding chemotherapy drugs in the peripheral nervous system: correlations with time course and neurotoxic severity. Cancer Res 2016;76:3332–9.

26. Gilardini A, Marmiroli P, Cavaletti G. Proteasome inhibition: a promising strategy for treating cancer, but what about neurotoxicity? Curr Med Chem 2008;15: 3025–35.

27. Casafont I, Berciano MT, Lafarga M. Bortezomib induces the formation of nuclear poly(A) RNA granules enriched in Sam68 and PABPN1 in sensory ganglia neurons. Neurotox Res 2010;17:167–78.

28. Bruna J, Udina E, Ale A, et al. Neurophysiological, histological and immunohistochemical characterization of bortezomib-induced neuropathy in mice. Exp Neurol 2010;223(2):599–608.

29. Chan ML, Stewart AK. Carfilzomib: a novel second-generation proteasome inhibitor. Future Oncol 2011;7:607–12.

30. Cardoso F, deAzambuja E, Lago LD. Current perspectives of epothilones in breast cancer. Eur J Cancer 2008;44:341–52.

31. Wozniak KM, Nomoto K, Lapidus RG, et al. Comparison of neuropathy-inducing effects of Eribulin Mesylate, Paclitaxel, and Ixabepilone in mice. Cancer Res 2011;71(11):3952–62.

32. Radomsky CL, Levine N. Thalidomide. Dermatol Clin 2001;19(1):87–103.

33. Park SB, Goldstein D, Krishnan AV, et al. Chemotherapy-induced peripheral neurotoxicity: a critical analysis. CA Cancer J Clin 2013;63:419–37.

34. Postma TJ, Aaronson NK, Heimans JJ, et al. The development of an EORTC quality of life questionnaire to assess chemotherapy-induced peripheral neuropathy: the QLQ-CIPN20. Eur J Cancer 2005;41(8):1135–9.

35. Oken MM, Creech RH, Tormey DC, et al. Toxicity and response criteria of the Eastern Cooperative Oncology Group. Am J Clin Oncol 1982;5:649–55.

36. Miller AB, Hoogstraten B, Staquet M, et al. Reporting results of cancer treatment. Cancer 1981;47:207–14.

37. Alberti P, Rossi E, Cornblath DR, et al. Physician-assessed and patient-reported outcome measures in chemotherapy-induced sensory peripheral neurotoxicity: two sides of the same coin. Ann Oncol 2014;25(1):257–64.

38. Brewer JR, Morrison G, Dolan ME, et al. Chemotherapy-induced peripheral neuropathy: current status and progress. Gynecol Oncol 2016;140:176–83.

39. Chaudhry V, Rowinsky EK, Sartorius SE, et al. Peripheral neuropathy from taxol and cisplatin combination chemotherapy: clinical and electrophysiological studies. Ann Neurol 1994;35:304–11.

40. Stubblefield MD, O'Dell MW. Electrodiagnosis in cancer. In: cancer rehabilitation: principles and practice. New York: Demos Medical; 2009. p. 649–67.

41. Krarup-Hansen A, Helweg-Larsen S, Schmalbruch H, et al. Neuronal involvement in cisplatin neuropathy: prospective clinical and neurophysiological studies. Brain 2007;130:1076–88.

42. Boehmerle W, Huehnchen P, Peruzzaro S, et al. Electrophysiological, behavioral and histological characterization of paclitaxel, cisplatin, vincristine and bortezomib-induced neuropathy in C57Bl/6 mice. Sci Rep 2014;4:6370.

43. Thompson SW, Davis LE, Kornfeld M, et al. Cisplatin neuropathy. Clinical, electrophysiologic, morphologic, and toxicologic studies. Cancer 1984;54:1269–75.

44. Boyette-Davis J, Dougherty PM. Protection against oxaliplatin-induced mechanical hyperalgesia and intraepidermal nerve fiber loss by minocycline. Exp Neurol 2011;229:353–7.

45. Argyriou AA, Koltzenburg M, Polychronopoulos P, et al. Peripheral nerve damage associated with administration of taxanes in patients with cancer. Crit Rev Oncol Hematol 2008;66:218–28.

46. Chen X, Stubblefield MD, Custodio CM, et al. Electrophysiological features of taxane-induced polyneuropathy in patients with breast cancer. J Clin Neurophysiol 2013;302:199–203.

47. Lersch C, Schmelz R, Eckel F, et al. Prevention of oxaliplatin-induced peripheral sensory neuropathy by carbamazepine in patients with advanced colorectal cancer. Clin Colorectal Cancer 2002;2:54–8.

48. Kassem LA, Yassin NA. Role of erythropoietin in prevention of chemotherapy-induced peripheral neuropathy. Pak J Biol Sci 2010;13:577–87.

49. Albers JW, Chaudhry V, Cavaletti G, et al. Interventions for preventing neuropathy caused by cisplatin and related compounds. Cochrane Database Syst Rev 2014;(3):CD005228.

50. Smith EM, Pang H, Cirrincione C, et al. Effect of duloxetine on pain, function, and quality of life among patients with chemotherapy-induced painful peripheral neuropathy: a randomized clinical trial. JAMA 2013;309(13):1359–67.

51. Stubblefield MD, O'Dell MW. Radiation fibrosis syndrome. In: cancer rehabilitation: principles and practice. New York: Demos Medical; 2009. p. 723–45.

52. Stubblefield MD. Clinical evaluation and management of radiation fibrosis syndrome. Phys Med Rehabil Clin N Am 2017;28(1):89–100.

53. Stubblefield MD. Radiation fibrosis syndrome: neuromuscular and musculoskeletal complications in cancer survivors. PM R 2011;3(11):1041–54.

54. Hauer-Jensen M, Fink LM, Wang J. Radiation injury and the protein C pathway. Crit Care Med 2004;32(5 Suppl):S325–30.

55. Delanian S, Lefaix JL. The radiation-induced fibroatrophic process: therapeutic perspective via the antioxidant pathway. Radiother Oncol 2004;73:119–31.

56. Trott K-R, Kamprad F. Radiobiological mechanisms of anti-inflammatory radiotherapy. Radiother Oncol 1999;51:197–203.

57. Denham J, Hauer-Jensen M. The radiotherapeutic injury—a complex 'wound'. Radiother Oncol 2002;63:129–45.

58. Nakamura K, Sasaki T, Ohga S, et al. Recent advances in radiation oncology: intensity-modulated radiotherapy, a clinical perspective. Int J Clin Oncol 2014;19(4):564–9.

59. Stubblefield MD, Ibanez K, Riedel ER, et al. Peripheral nervous system injury after high-dose single fraction image-guided sterotactic radiosurgery for spine tumors. Neurosurg Focus 2017;42(3):E12.

60. Qui WZ, Peng XS, Xia HQ, et al. A retrospective study comparing the outcomes and toxicities of intensity-modulated radiotherapy versus two-dimensional conventional radiotherapy for the treatment of children and adolescent nasopharyngeal carcinoma. J Cancer Res Clin Oncol 2017;143(8):1563–72.

61. Stubblefield MD, Burstein HJ, Burton AW, et al. NCCN task force report: management of neuropathy in cancer. J Natl Compr Canc Netw 2009;7(Suppl 5):S1–26 [quiz: S27–8].

62. Okereke LI, Custodio CM, Stubblefield MD. Bilateral lower-trunk brachial plexopathy and proximal myopathy 19 years after mantle field radiation for Hodgkin's disease: a case report. Arch Phys Med Rehabil 2004;85:e23–4.

63. Stout NL, Silver JK, Raj VS, et al. Toward a national initiative in cancer rehabilitation: recommendations from a subject matter expert group. Arch Phys Med Rehabil 2016;97(11):2006–15.
64. Stubblefield MD, Levien A, Custodio CM, et al. The role of botulinum toxin type A in the radiation fibrosis syndrome: a preliminary report. Arch Phys Med Rehabil 2008;89(3):417–21.

Predicting Recovery from Peripheral Nerve Trauma

Lawrence R. Robinson, MD

KEYWORDS

- Electrodiagnosis • Prognosis • Focal neuropathy • Traumatic neuropathy
- Outcome

KEY POINTS

- Prognosis of focal nerve injuries is an important piece of information for those managing these types of patients.
- By providing an estimate of outcome from a nerve injury, one allows the treating physician to make an informed recommendation regarding treatment options.
- For those with a poor prognosis for spontaneous recovery, tendon transfers may be a good early option or, in some cases, early nerve transfers or grafting may be indicated.
- A patient with a good prognosis for recovery may be better treated conservatively, because spontaneous recovery is usually better than surgical treatment.

INTRODUCTION

The prognosis for focal nerve injuries is an important piece of information for those managing these types of patients. By providing an estimate of outcome from a nerve injury, one allows the treating physician to make an informed recommendation regarding treatment options. For those with a poor prognosis for spontaneous recovery, tendon transfers may be a good early option or, in some cases, early nerve transfers or grafting may be indicated. In contrast, a patient with a good prognosis for recovery may be better treated conservatively, because spontaneous recovery is usually better than surgical treatment.

In this article, we discuss the types of nerve injuries that have better prognoses, review which electrodiagnostic measures are generally useful for predicting outcome, and summarize the information available for focal injuries of the commonly affected and studied nerves so that nerve-specific information can be provided. We also discuss the challenges in using electrodiagnostic data to predict prognosis.

Disclosure: The author has nothing to disclose.
Physical Medicine and Rehabilitation, University of Toronto, Sunnybrook Health Sciences Centre, H391, 2075 Bayview Avenue, Toronto, Ontario M4N 3M5, Canada
E-mail address: Larry.Robinson@Sunnybrook.ca

Phys Med Rehabil Clin N Am 29 (2018) 721–733
https://doi.org/10.1016/j.pmr.2018.06.007
1047-9651/18/© 2018 Elsevier Inc. All rights reserved.
pmr.theclinics.com

Abbreviations	
BR	Brachioradialis
CFN	Common fibular nerve
CMAP	Compound muscle action potential
CTS	Carpal tunnel syndrome
EDB	Extensor digitorum brevis
MCP	Metacarpophalangeal
MUAP	Motor unit action potential
PACN	Posterior antebrachial cutaneous nerve
ROM	Range of motion
SNAP	Sensory nerve action potential
TA	Tibialis anterior

GRADING OF TRAUMATIC NERVE INJURY

Traumatic peripheral nerve injuries can be classified according to the degree of disruption of axons and their supporting structures.[1] This classification represents a significant determinant of outcome. Seddon defined 3 grades of classification: (1) neurapraxia, (2) axonotmesis, and (3) neurotmesis.[2]

Neurapraxia is a primarily demyelinating injury that has a good prognosis, because most patients experience recovery within 2 to 3 months as remyelination occurs and conduction block resolves.[2] In axonotmesis, there is disruption of axons with at least partial preservation of supporting structures, such as the perineurium (surrounding fascicles) or epineurium (the outer covering of the nerve). Axonotmetic injuries have variable prognosis depending on the ability of axons to regrow. Nerve injuries with more severe disruption of supporting elements of the nerve will have a lower chance of recovery than those with minimal disruption.[3] In injuries with extensive disruption of the fascicular structure and local scarring and fibrosis, there is a lesser chance of axons growing through the region of injury and reaching their end organs on the other side. Similarly, neuroma formation at the site of injury makes it unlikely that axons will make it through the neuroma and across the injury site to fulfill their destined function. Finally in neurotmesis, there is complete disruption of both the axons and the supporting structures of the nerve and there is little chance of recovery without surgical intervention.

DEGREE OF DEMYELINATION

The extent of demyelination may also influence recovery, but this seems to have less impact than the degree of axon loss. Severe disruption of myelin can certainly produce conduction block and clinical deficits. But after a loss of myelin, Schwann cells generally have the capacity to remyelinate demyelinated areas of the nerve, and conduction improves. The morphology and function of the myelin will not be the same as before the injury,[4] and slowed conduction velocity may persist.[5] Nevertheless, because of the capacity for remyelination, in general neurapraxic traumatic nerve injury has a good prognosis, with the majority of patients experiencing substantial recovery within 2 to 3 months.

EXTENT OF AXON LOSS

The degree of axon loss has a large impact on prognosis. Nerve injuries with minimal axon loss generally have a better prognosis. When some motor axons are spared, fortunately they have the capacity to reinnervate some denervated muscle fibers by distal axon sprouting. Thus, this process can accommodate relatively mild degrees of axon loss even if no axons regrow from the site of the injury. Human motor axons can reinnervate about 5 times their original muscle fiber territory by this process[6]; hence, even substantial axon loss can recover without axon regrowth. However, when the great majority of axons are lost (eg, >90%), the small number of surviving axons cannot expand their territory sufficiently to produce the strength needed for full function.

DISTANCE TO THE MUSCLE

When axons need to grow from the site of nerve injury for recovery to occur, the distance from the injury site to the muscle has an important impact on prognosis. In axonotmetic injuries in which the endoneural tubes are preserved, the axons can traverse the segment of injury in 1 to 2 weeks and regenerate along the distal nerve segment at a rate of 1 to 5 mm/d[3]; this is faster proximally and in younger individuals.[7] When the distance is short, axons can reach muscle fibers while the axon tubes are still capable of accommodating regrowth and before axonal stenosis occurs and prevents reinnervation. The muscle will still be viable and open to reinnervation. However, in severe injuries with complete or near-complete loss of motor axons, after approximately 18 months the muscle can no longer be reinnervated, even if the axons reach it.[8] The axon tubes will be stenotic, the muscle may be fibrotic, and contractures may have formed. Thus, in complete axon loss injuries with long distances to reinnervate, such as lower trunk brachial plexus injuries, the prognosis is poor even if fascicular disruption is minimal.[9]

WHICH ELECTRODIAGNOSTIC MEASURES ARE GENERALLY USEFUL FOR ESTIMATING PROGNOSIS?
Compound Muscle Action Potential Amplitude

Compound muscle action potential (CMAP) amplitude is a useful method for estimating the extent of axon loss or axon preservation. CMAP amplitude is roughly proportional to the number of excitable motor axons. Thus, when stimulating distal to the injury site and recording from the supplied muscle, the CMAP amplitude gives an estimate of the degree of axonal preservation. If one stimulates proximal to the injury, however, the CMAP is also influenced by the extent of demyelination and conduction block (**Fig. 1**).

When conduction block is observed in peripheral nerve injuries, this sign is actually good. Conduction block, when observed after the first week after injury, is only seen in demyelinating injuries. Because these injuries have a greater capacity to recover than axon loss injuries, the presence of conduction block is generally favorable.

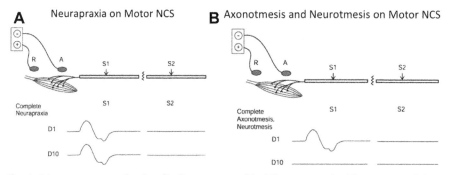

Fig. 1. Motor nerve conduction findings expected in (*A*) neurapraxia, (*B*) axonotmesis/neurotmesis, at days 1 and 10 after injury.

Although generally useful, there are limitations to using the distal CMAP for estimating the number of axons. Acutely, it can take up to 7 days for the CMAP to diminish in size or disappear.[10,11] Hence, using this measure too early can provide misleading results and overestimate the number of viable axons.

Beginning several months after injury, the CMAP amplitude can also overestimate the number of axons that are preserved. Once sufficient time has passed for distal axon sprouting to occur, typically 2 to 3 months, each axon will supply more than its typical number of motor axons. When stimulated, each axon will produce a larger motor unit action potential (MUAP) and when the whole nerve is stimulated a larger CMAP will be produced. One then can overestimate the number of excitable motor axons. Because the larger CMAP is recorded after axon sprouting has occurred, there is no longer the same unused capacity for reinnervation. Hence a CMAP that is 30% of normal at 1 month after injury is a better sign than the same size CMAP at 1 year after injury.

Another limitation of using the CMAP for estimating prognosis relates to which muscle is used for recording. Ideally, one should record from a functionally important muscle, such as the tibialis anterior (TA) in the case of fibular neuropathy rather than from the extensor digitorum brevis (EDB). Despite these limitations, CMAP amplitude is an important measure of axon loss, injury severity, and ultimately prognosis.

Sensory Nerve Action Potential Amplitude

The sensory nerve action potential (SNAP) amplitude is a reflection of the number of excitable sensory axons. Patients with preserved sensory amplitude sometimes have a less severe injury and better sensory outcomes.[12,13] However, SNAP amplitudes are less useful than CMAP amplitudes. SNAPs are smaller and more challenging to record than CMAPs. In addition, motor strength may play a more obvious role in functional recovery than sensation.

Nerve Conduction Velocity

Slowing of nerve conduction velocity is primarily a reflection of the extent of demyelination of the nerve, although nerve conduction velocity is also influenced by the loss of larger diameter axons. As noted, demyelination has less impact on prognosis than axon loss. Hence, nerve conduction velocity is not a strong predictor of recovery. Slowing may actually be a good predictor of outcome,[14] because those with impairments resulting from demyelination are more likely to recover than those with deficits owing to axon loss.

Needle Electromyography: Spontaneous Activity

With motor axon loss, fibrillation potentials and positive sharp waves appear after 10 to 14 days in muscles closer to the injury site and after 3 to 4 weeks in more distal muscles. These potentials are recorded in the presence of even small degrees of axon loss and are typically graded on an ordinal scale from 1+ (reproducible potentials in >1 area) to 4+ (obliterating the baseline). Higher grades represent more axon loss than lower grades. However, the presence and density of fibrillations and positive sharp waves do not significantly impact prognosis, either in focal or generalized neuropathies.[12,15,16]

There are several reasons for the lack of association between fibrillations and positive sharp waves and outcome. First, the grading scheme is an ordinal scale, not a ratio or interval scale. Thus, 2+ positive sharp waves likely represent more axon loss than 1+, but not necessarily twice as much; we do not know how much more. Additionally, it may be that loss of a relatively small proportion of the total axons can result in 4+ fibrillations.[17]

Needle Electromyography Recruitment

Voluntary MUAP recruitment on needle electromyography can be useful to establish the presence of intact motor axons under voluntary control and can provide a rough indication of the degree of axon preservation. This measure is especially useful for examining the muscles immediately distal to the injury site. The presence of MUAP recruitment in these proximal muscles indicates that the injury is not complete and that at least some axons are successfully traversing the injury site and exciting muscle fibers on the other side. When recruitment is normal or only mildly reduced in a muscle innervated just distal to the injury site, this is an important favorable prognostic factor that may be as important as, or more important than, CMAP amplitude.[15]

At the same time, recruitment has limitations as a prognostic measure. It is difficult to quantify and is usually recorded on a subjective ordinal scale, such as full, reduced, discrete, or none. In addition, poor or absent recruitment does not indicate unequivocal axon loss; conduction block can produce similar findings.

General Prognostic Features

The generally favorable versus unfavorable prognostic factors can be seen in **Table 1**. This is a good starting point to keep in mind for most cases. For a more accurate prognosis, however, it is likely better to use nerve specific information when possible (**Table 2**).

HOW MUCH VARIABILITY IS THERE BETWEEN NERVES?

In addition to the general principles of how one might use electrodiagnostic measures to establish prognosis, there is considerable variability between different nerves in the limbs and face. The variability limits extrapolation and requires one to customize the assessment to each nerve.

First, there are anatomic variables that influence the prognosis of individual focal nerve lesions. Distance is a significant factor. Shorter nerves have a limited distance to grow to resupply muscles, such as the facial nerve, and they have different challenges than those with longer distances, such as proximal ulnar or sciatic nerve lesions. As discussed elsewhere in this article, muscle may remain viable for about 18 months after denervation and hence muscles distant from the site of a severe nerve injury will have lower chances of recovery than those with shorter distances to cover.

For cranial nerves in particular, synkinesis can be a limiting factor in recovery and can be problematic for injuries to the facial or laryngeal nerves.[18,19] After disruptive injuries to these nerves, axons can regrow from the site of injury but grow in the "wrong"

Table 1		
Generally useful prognostic measures for focal peripheral nerve injuries		
Useful Prognostic Factors	**Good Prognosis**	**Poor Prognosis**
Recruitment of muscle distal to injury	Normal or reduced	Discrete or absent
Distal CMAP	Normal or reduced	Absent
Conduction block or slowing	Present	Absent
Distal SNAP (for injuries distal to the DRG)	Present	Absent
Distal SNAP (for root avulsions)		Present

These factors are most useful after 7 days, but within the first 2 to 3 months after injury, before reinnervation by collateral sprouting has been substantial.

Abbreviations: CMAP, compound muscle action potential; DRG, dorsal root ganglion; SNAP, sensory nerve action potential.

Table 2
Best and worst prognostic groups for specific nerve injuries

Nerve	Best Prognostic Group	Poor Prognosis
Median	SNAPs present CSI 2.5–4.6 Motor latency of <6.5 ms	Normal study Absent CMAPs and SNAPs
Ulnar	Conduction block or slowing across the elbow; normal CMAP amplitudes	Small or absent CMAP, no conduction block
Radial	BR recruitment reduced or normal	BR recruitment absent or discrete Absent CMAP to extensor indicis
Fibular	TA and EDB CMAP present	TA and EDB CMAP absent
Facial	CMAP of >%30 of contralateral side Presence of blink reflex	CMAP of <10% of contralateral side

Abbreviations: BR, brachioradialis; CMAP, compound muscle action potential; CSI, combined sensory index; EDB, extensor digitorum brevis; SNAP, sensory nerve action potential; TA, tibialis anterior.

neural tubes and supply different muscles than their original destination. This regrowth might not produce functional recovery and can even result in more dysfunction than if regrowth did not occur at all. In contrast, synkinesis is generally not a problem in limb nerves and muscles.

The function and functional requirements of each nerve are also variable. The facial nerve requires fine, precise control with relatively little force, as does the laryngeal nerve. In contrast, the femoral nerve does not require particularly fine control, but needs to produce sufficient knee extensor strength for weightbearing and functional ambulation. Different segments of each nerve may play more or less critical roles in function. For the ulnar nerve, innervation of proximal muscles, such as flexor carpi ulnaris or flexor digitorum profundus, are helpful, but innervation of distal hand muscles is more critical for functional recovery. However, for the fibular nerve, the proximally innervated TA and fibularis longus are important for function, whereas distal muscles play a much smaller role; here, just a few centimeters of reinnervation may be sufficient for a good outcome.

Although muscle strength is more straightforward to quantify, sensation plays a very important role in functional recovery for some nerves. The median nerve sensory supply covers the majority of the hand and, without adequate sensation, even with good motor strength, it would be difficult to use the hand to its full capacity. In contrast, some nerves such as the anterior interosseous nerve have no cutaneous sensation, and others, such as the deep fibular have limited sensory distributions.

The mechanism and pathophysiology of injury also varies between nerves. The median nerve is most commonly affected by distal entrapment at the carpal tunnel, which is a predominantly demyelinating injury. In contrast, the ulnar nerve tends to have a substantial frequency of axon loss, even in chronic compressive lesions.[20] The radial and sciatic nerves are rarely entrapped by chronic ongoing compression, but are commonly affected by traumatic injury of the upper and lower limbs, respectively.[21] Each of these mechanisms of injury potentially carries a different likelihood of a good outcome and the prognosis may be different even with similar electrodiagnostic measures (**Fig. 2**).

Not only does natural history vary considerably between nerves, but so do treatment options. For some nerves, there are good treatment options even if the nerve does not regenerate. In the setting of radial neuropathy, tendon transfers can produce a reasonably good functional outcome even in the absence of strength recovery in radial

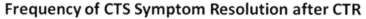

Frequency of CTS Symptom Resolution after CTR

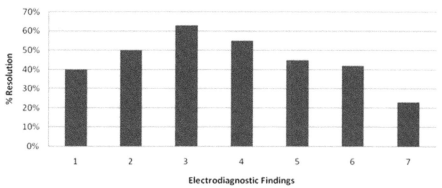

Electrodiagnostic Criteria	Frequency
1. Normal study	40%
2. CSI 1.0 – 2.5	50%
3. CSI 2.5 – 4.6	63%
4. CSI > 4.6, Sensory responses present	55%
5. Sensories absent, motor latency <6.5 ms	45%
6. Motor latency >6.5ms	42%
7. Absent motor and sensory responses	23%

Fig. 2. Prognostic information on the likelihood of complete symptom resolution in patients with carpal tunnel syndrome (CTS) if they undergo carpal tunnel release. CSI, combined sensory index.

innervated muscles. Custom fabricated ankle foot orthoses can compensate for ankle dorsiflexor weakness in fibular neuropathy. There are fewer good options, however, for severe brachial plexopathies or complete median or ulnar nerve lesions.

Median Nerve

Electrodiagnostic studies, primarily nerve conduction studies, offer some ability to predict outcome after carpal tunnel release surgery.[22–26] It seems from these studies that those with moderate nerve conduction study abnormalities have the greatest likelihood of achieving good relief of symptoms after surgery, whereas those with relatively normal studies, or those with marked abnormalities, have a lower chance of relief.

Bland[22] has reported that those with normal studies and those with more severe changes (motor latencies of >6.5 ms) had only about a 40% chance of complete symptom resolution, whereas those with moderate changes between the 2 extremes did considerably better. A similar finding was reported by Malladi and colleagues[23] using the Combined Sensory Index as the nerve conduction study variable.[27]

Ulnar Nerve

The 2 most important measures that predict a good outcome for patients with ulnar neuropathy at the elbow are preserved CMAP amplitude in ulnar hand muscles and the presence of conduction block and slowing across the elbow.[12,14,20,28] In 1 study,[12] overall subjective recovery was best predicted by the combination of the presence of conduction block to the first dorsal interosseous muscle and normal distal abductor digiti minimi CMAP amplitude; 87% of patients recovered if the combination of conduction block and normal CMAP was present, whereas only 7% recovered who did not meet either criterion. The authors of this study reported that these 2 variables, taken together, produce a greater degree of separation of outcomes than any single variable alone (**Fig. 3**).[18] Other studies have also reported that the presence of a conduction block or slowing (indicating demyelination) is suggestive of a good outcome.[14,28] There is little in the literature to suggest that needle electromyography findings play a significant role in an accurate prognosis. A recent study has proposed a prognostic estimation framework that includes clinical, electrodiagnostic, and ultrasound findings.[29] An unfavorable outcome was associated with right-sided ulnar neuropathy at the elbow, more severe weakness of the abductor digiti minimi, and more pronounced ulnar nerve thickening on ultrasound. A CMAP reduction across the elbow of 16% or greater was associated with a more favorable outcome.

Radial Nerve

Electrodiagnosis can provide important information for determining outcome after radial nerve injury. In 1 study,[15] the most useful prognostic indicators were recruitment in the brachioradialis (BR) and CMAP amplitude recorded from the extensor indicis. When recruitment in the BR was full, 100% had a good outcome, even if distal muscles had poor recruitment. In addition, 80% of those with discrete recruitment (reduced numbers of rapidly firing MUAPs) in BR did well, whereas only 38% of those with absent recruitment in BR had a good outcome. CMAP amplitude from the extensor indicis contributed to the estimation of prognosis, but less so than recruitment. The presence of MUAP recruitment in BR is important because it demonstrates that some axons are traversing the injury site and that there is a pathway for others to

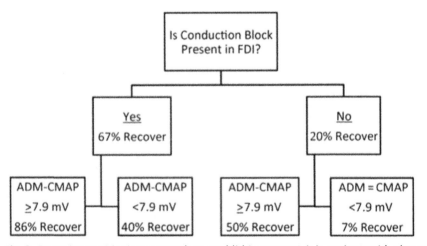

Fig. 3. Recursive partitioning approach to establishing prognosis in patients with ulnar neuropathy. ADM-CMAP, abductor digiti minimi-compound muscle action potential; FDI, first dorsal interosseous.

establish reinnervation to distal muscles. As with other examples, the density of fibrillation potentials has not been shown to be correlated with outcomes after radial neuropathy. Just as for the ulnar nerve, combining 2 variables (recruitment and CMAP amplitude) seems to offer more separation into prognostic groups than using a single variable alone (**Fig. 4**). Another study looking at outcomes in nontraumatic radial neuropathies used multiple logistic regression analysis to find that conduction block on nerve conduction studies, younger age, and less severe initial weakness are indicators for a good prognosis.[30]

Fibular Nerve

The fibular nerve (formerly known by some as the peroneal nerve or lateral popliteal nerve[31]) is the most commonly injured peripheral nerve in the lower extremity when injuries to the fibular division of the sciatic nerve are included.[32] When assessing prognosis for fibular nerve injuries, it is important to carefully consider which muscles to evaluate. Although the distal EDB is commonly used for fibular motor nerve conduction study, this muscle contributes little to function. Thus, it is often helpful to record from the more functionally important TA when performing motor nerve conduction studies of this nerve.

There have been a number of studies of which electrodiagnostic measures are most useful for assessment of prognosis. One study[33] combined nerve conduction study of the TA and the EDB with recruitment data and showed a linear relationship between CMAP amplitude and outcome (**Fig. 5**). Of those with a normal CMAP to the TA, 92% had a good outcome, whereas only 46% of those with an absent CMAP did well. This study also demonstrated that additional useful information was obtained by recording from both EDB and TA, as opposed to recording from only a single muscle. Similarly, in a series of patients with common fibular mononeuropathy, Katirji and

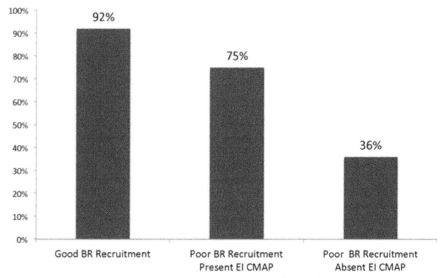

Fig. 4. Percent of patients who achieve good recovery after radial nerve injury. Group 1: recruitment full, central, or reduced; compound muscle action potential (CMAP) present or absent. Group 2: recruitment discrete or none; CMAP present. Group 3: recruitment discrete or none; CMAP absent. BR, brachioradialis; EI, extensor indicis.

Fibular Nerve - Percentage of subjects with good recovery based on CMAP amplitude.

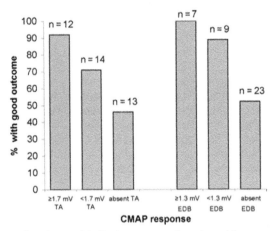

Fig. 5. Percent of patients with fibular neuropathy who achieve a good outcome, based on compound muscle action potential (CMAP) amplitude in tibialis anterior (TA; *left 3 bars*) and extensor digitorum brevis (EDB; *right 3 bars*).

Wilbourn[34] showed that axon loss was substantial in 80% of cases and that TA CMAP amplitude may be best suited to assess the severity of the injury. As with radial neuropathy, Bsteh and colleagues[30] reported that a good outcome is predicted by younger age, greater strength on initial evaluation, and the presence of conduction block on nerve conduction studies.

Facial Nerve

With respect to electrodiagnostic estimation of prognosis in facial neuropathy, it has been demonstrated that CMAP amplitude is the most important metric. Patients with CMAP amplitudes of 30% or greater of the opposite side have an excellent outcome, those with amplitudes of 10% to 30% have a good but not always complete recovery, and those with an amplitude of less than 10% have a poor outcome.[35] This finding has often been used by otolaryngologists to determine the need for surgical intervention. More recent studies have found different cutoffs to be useful. In a study of 120 subjects, Mancini and colleagues[36] reported that amplitudes of less than 23% of the unaffected sided were the strongest predictor of nonrecovery of normal function. Using receiver operating curve analysis, the strongest prediction values of amplitude compared with the contralateral side were 33% (67% sensitivity, 81% specificity) and 45% (100% sensitivity, 68% specificity) at baseline and second evaluations, respectively; amplitudes below these values were associated with a poor prognosis.

The timing of electrodiagnostic assessment plays an important role in evaluation of facial nerve injuries. Especially in the setting of temporal bone fracture, the timing of changes seen on facial motor nerve conduction studies impacts the prognosis of facial nerve injuries. Studying the nerve too early—before the occurrence of Wallerian degeneration (ie, before day 7)—will falsely lead to the conclusion that more axons are viable than there really are. In contrast, waiting too long could result in missed opportunities for early surgical intervention. Generally, studies between days 7 and 14 after onset are preferable.[37]

In terms of outcome after temporal bone fracture, those with less severe injuries have a good spontaneous return of function, including those with a less than 95% decrease in the CMAP in the first 14 days.[38–40] Poorer outcomes have been noted for patients with a greater than 95% degeneration in CMAP within 14 days of injury and these patients are routinely offered surgical decompression.

Brachial Plexus

Brachial plexus injuries occur in roughly 2% to 3% of all admissions to level I trauma hospitals.[21] Most commonly, they result from car or motorcycle crashes, or motor vehicle versus pedestrian accidents.[41] A key prognostic element in the evaluation of brachial plexus injuries is the determination of whether there has been an avulsion of 1 or more of the roots from the spinal cord. This factor is critical because nerve root avulsions do not recover and performing plexus surgery distal to a root avulsion is generally pointless.[9,42] The 2 primary ways to evaluate for root avulsion are by studying SNAPs and paraspinal muscles. When SNAPs are present in the face of severe limb denervation, this finding suggests that the injury may be proximal to the dorsal root ganglion, that is, root avulsion. When SNAPs are absent or markedly decreased, this finding indicates a more distal injury, but it does not necessarily indicate that the root is intact, because root avulsion and plexus injuries can coexist as a result of severe trauma. The presence of abnormalities in the paraspinal muscles also suggests root avulsion, or at least that the injury has occurred proximal to the division of the posterior primary ramus from the spinal nerve root.

The prognosis of brachial plexus injuries is also affected by the site of injury. Kim and colleagues[43] studied the outcomes of 1,019 surgically managed brachial plexus injuries. Outcomes were best when injuries involved the upper and middle trunks, primarily supplied by the C5, C6, and C7 roots, or the lateral or posterior cords, but poor for C8 or T1 root injuries, lower trunk injuries, or medial cord involvement. The distance required for reinnervation of muscles supplied by the lower plexus likely plays a role in the poorer prognosis. Complete injuries of the plexus have a very poor prognosis.[44] It is possible that a reason for a relatively good prognosis in upper trunk and middle trunk injuries is that these segments of the plexus innervate proximal muscles with relatively short distances for axonal regrowth. Moreover, these muscles supply robust proximal arm motions only, in contrast with the fine hand movements that are generally related to lower and middle trunk innervation.

SUMMARY

Providing a prognosis for patients with focal peripheral nerve injuries is an important component of the electrodiagnostic medical consultation. There are a variety of electrodiagnostic measures that may provide valuable prognostic information. Although there are some generally useful principles to apply to most nerve injuries, the interpretation should be individualized for each nerve and clinical context. Future research should focus on prospective studies to provide additional insight into the factors that enhance the accuracy of outcome prediction.

REFERENCES

1. Robinson LR. Traumatic injury to peripheral nerves. Muscle Nerve 2000;23(6): 863–73.

2. Seddon H. Surgical disorders of the peripheral nerves. 2nd edition. New York: Churchill Livingstone; 1975. p. 336.
3. Sunderland S. Nerves and nerve injuries. 2nd edition. New York: Churchill Livingstone ; distributed by Longman; 1978. p. 1046.
4. Fowler TJ, Danta G, Gilliatt RW. Recovery of nerve conduction after a pneumatic tourniquet: observations on the hind-limb of the baboon. J Neurol Neurosurg Psychiatry 1972;35(5):638–47.
5. Melvin JL, Johnson EW, Duran R. Electrodiagnosis after surgery for the carpal tunnel syndrome. Arch Phys Med Rehabil 1968;49(9):502–7.
6. Brown MC, Holland RL, Hopkins WG. Motor nerve sprouting. Annu Rev Neurosci 1981;4:17–42.
7. Burnett MG, Zager EL. Pathophysiology of peripheral nerve injury: a brief review. Neurosurg Focus 2004;16(5):E1.
8. Gutmann E, Young JZ. The re-innervation of muscle after various periods of atrophy. J Anat 1944;78(Pt 1–2):15–43.
9. Campbell WW. Evaluation and management of peripheral nerve injury. Clin Neurophysiol 2008;119(9):1951–65.
10. Chaudhry V, Cornblath DR. Wallerian degeneration in human nerves: serial electrophysiological studies. Muscle Nerve 1992;15(6):687–93.
11. Gilliatt RW, Hjorth RJ. Nerve conduction during Wallerian degeneration in the balloon. J Neurol Neurosurg Psychiatry 1972;35(3):335–41.
12. Friedrich JM, Robinson LR. Prognostic indicators from electrodiagnostic studies for ulnar neuropathy at the elbow. Muscle Nerve 2011;43(4):596–600.
13. Lo YL, Prakash KM, Leoh TH, et al. Posterior antebrachial cutaneous nerve conduction study in radial neuropathy. J Neurol Sci 2004;223(2):199–202.
14. Beekman R, Wokke JH, Schoemaker MC, et al. Ulnar neuropathy at the elbow: follow-up and prognostic factors determining outcome. Neurology 2004;63(9): 1675–80.
15. Malikowski T, Micklesen PJ, Robinson LR. Prognostic values of electrodiagnostic studies in traumatic radial neuropathy. Muscle Nerve 2007;36(3):364–7.
16. Miller RG, Peterson GW, Daube JR, et al. Prognostic value of electrodiagnosis in Guillain-Barre syndrome. Muscle Nerve 1988;11(7):769–74.
17. Dumitru D, Amato AA, Zwarts MJ. Electrodiagnostic medicine. 2nd edition. Philadelphia: Hanley & Belfus; 2002. p. xi, 1524.
18. Maronian NC, Robinson L, Waugh P, et al. A new electromyographic definition of laryngeal synkinesis. Ann Otol Rhinol Laryngol 2004;113(11):877–86.
19. Valls-Sole J, Montero J. Movement disorders in patients with peripheral facial palsy. Mov Disord 2003;18(12):1424–35.
20. Beekman R, Van Der Plas JP, Uitdehaag BM, et al. Clinical, electrodiagnostic, and sonographic studies in ulnar neuropathy at the elbow. Muscle Nerve 2004; 30(2):202–8.
21. Noble J, Munro CA, Prasad VS, et al. Analysis of upper and lower extremity peripheral nerve injuries in a population of patients with multiple injuries. J Trauma 1998;45(1):116–22.
22. Bland JD. Do nerve conduction studies predict the outcome of carpal tunnel decompression? Muscle Nerve 2001;24(7):935–40.
23. Malladi N, Micklesen PJ, Hou J, et al. Correlation between the combined sensory index and clinical outcome after carpal tunnel decompression: a retrospective review. Muscle Nerve 2010;41(4):453–7.
24. Rigler I, Podnar S. Impact of electromyographic findings on choice of treatment and outcome. Eur J Neurol 2007;14(7):783–7.

25. Jarvik JG, Comstock BA, Heagerty PJ, et al. Magnetic resonance imaging compared with electrodiagnostic studies in patients with suspected carpal tunnel syndrome: predicting symptoms, function, and surgical benefit at 1 year. J Neurosurg 2008;108(3):541–50.

26. Lo YL, Lim SH, Fook-Chong S, et al. Outcome prediction value of nerve conduction studies for endoscopic carpal tunnel surgery. J Clin Neuromuscul Dis 2012; 13(3):153–8.

27. Robinson LR, Micklesen PJ, Wang L. Strategies for analyzing nerve conduction data: superiority of a summary index over single tests. Muscle Nerve 1998; 21(9):1166–71.

28. Dunselman HH, Visser LH. The clinical, electrophysiological and prognostic heterogeneity of ulnar neuropathy at the elbow. J Neurol Neurosurg Psychiatry 2008; 79(12):1364–7.

29. Beekman R, Zijlstra W, Visser LH. A novel points system to predict the prognosis of ulnar neuropathy at the elbow. Muscle Nerve 2017;55(5):698–705.

30. Bsteh G, Wanschitz JV, Gruber H, et al. Prognosis and prognostic factors in non-traumatic acute-onset compressive mononeuropathies–radial and peroneal mononeuropathies. Eur J Neurol 2013;20(6):981–5.

31. Robinson LR 2nd. What do we call that structure? Muscle Nerve 2010;42(6):981 [author reply: 981].

32. Robinson LR. Traumatic injury to peripheral nerves. Suppl Clin Neurophysiol 2004;57:173–86.

33. Derr JJ, Micklesen PJ, Robinson LR. Predicting recovery after fibular nerve injury: which electrodiagnostic features are most useful? Am J Phys Med Rehabil 2009; 88(7):547–53.

34. Katirji MB, Wilbourn AJ. Common peroneal mononeuropathy: a clinical and electrophysiologic study of 116 lesions. Neurology 1988;38(11):1723–8.

35. Sillman JS, Niparko JK, Lee SS, et al. Prognostic value of evoked and standard electromyography in acute facial paralysis. Otolaryngol Head Neck Surg 1992; 107(3):377–81.

36. Mancini P, De Seta D, Prosperini L, et al. Prognostic factors of Bell's palsy: multivariate analysis of electrophysiological findings. Laryngoscope 2014;124(11): 2598–605.

37. Claflin ES, Robinson LR. How soon after temporal bone fracture should we perform electroneurography? Muscle Nerve 2011;44(2):304.

38. Fisch U. Management of intratemporal facial nerve injuries. J Laryngol Otol 1980; 94(1):129–34.

39. Fisch U. Prognostic value of electrical tests in acute facial paralysis. Am J Otol 1984;5(6):494–8.

40. Chang CY, Cass SP. Management of facial nerve injury due to temporal bone trauma. Am J Otol 1999;20(1):96–114.

41. Midha R. Epidemiology of brachial plexus injuries in a multitrauma population. Neurosurgery 1997;40(6):1182–8 [discussion: 1188–9].

42. Terzis JK, Kostopoulos VK. The surgical treatment of brachial plexus injuries in adults. Plast Reconstr Surg 2007;119(4):73e–92e.

43. Kim DH, Cho YJ, Tiel RL, et al. Outcomes of surgery in 1019 brachial plexus lesions treated at Louisiana State University Health Sciences Center. J Neurosurg 2003;98(5):1005–16.

44. Rorabeck CH, Harris WR. Factors affecting the prognosis of brachial plexus injuries. J Bone Joint Surg Br 1981;63-B(3):404–7.

Electrodiagnosis in the Patient with Metabolic Syndrome: Adding Value to Patient Care

Karen P. Barr, MD

KEYWORDS

- Electrodiagnosis • Nerve conduction studies • Metabolic syndrome • Prediabetes
- Polyneuropathy • Carpal tunnel syndrome • Radiculopathy

KEY POINTS

- Patients with metabolic syndrome are at increased risk for peripheral neuropathy, entrapment neuropathy, and radiculopathy, even if they have normal blood glucose levels.
- Electrodiagnostic studies are often necessary in this population because of the complexity of their symptoms and overlapping conditions.
- Patients with metabolic syndrome are at risk for functional decline if their nerve disease is not addressed.

INTRODUCTION

Metabolic syndrome is a group of related conditions that includes impaired glucose metabolism, central obesity, hypertension, and hyperlipidemia (**Table 1** for diagnostic criteria). It is a common condition encountered in the electrodiagnostic laboratory because it has a high prevalence in the population and because patients with metabolic syndrome are prone to multiple peripheral nerve disorders.

The prevalence of metabolic syndrome has been increasing in the United States, and it is currently estimated that more than 35% of the US population has this disorder. It is particularly prevalent among older patients, with those older than age 70 having a five times higher risk than those younger than age 40.[1]

There is a well-known link between increased blood sugar and neuropathy.[2] An increasing body of evidence shows a link between other aspects of the metabolic syndrome and various neuropathies.[3] Patients with metabolic syndrome, even those without blood sugar dysfunction, have an increased risk of length-dependent

Disclosure Statement: Nothing to disclose.
Division of Physical Medicine and Rehabilitation, Department of Orthopaedics, West Virginia University, Box 9100, 1 Medical Center Drive, Morgantown, WV 26506, USA
E-mail address: Karen.barr@hsc.wvu.edu

Phys Med Rehabil Clin N Am 29 (2018) 735–749
https://doi.org/10.1016/j.pmr.2018.06.008
pmr.theclinics.com
1047-9651/18/© 2018 Elsevier Inc. All rights reserved.

Table 1
Diagnostic criteria for metabolic syndrome: three or more of the following

Criterion	Definition	Men	Women
Abdominal obesity	Waist circumference	≥40 in	≥35 in
Dyslipidemia[a]	Triglyceride level	≥150 mg/dL	Same
	Reduced high-density lipoprotein cholesterol	<40 mg/dL	<50 mg/dL
Hypertension[a]	Systolic or diastolic	≥130/85	Same
Hyperglycemia[a]	Fasting plasma glucose	≥100	Same

[a] Or taking medication to treat this condition.

Data from Grundy SM, Cleeman JI, Daniels SR, et al. Diagnosis and management of the metabolic syndrome: an American Heart Association/National Heart, Lung, and Blood Institute Scientific Statement. Circulation 2005;112(17):2735–52.

polyneuropathy, entrapment neuropathies, and radiculopathy.[4–7] A well-designed electrodiagnostic study can give information about these conditions that cannot be obtained any other way.

PATHOPHYSIOLOGY OF NERVE DAMAGE IN METABOLIC SYNDROME
Hyperglycemia

There is a well-established link between hyperglycemia and microvascular damage that causes neuropathy. Types of neuropathies linked to hyperglycemia include distal symmetric sensorimotor polyneuropathy (DPN), autonomic neuropathy, proximal neuropathies, focal neuropathies, and small fiber neuropathies. Neurons are at risk of damage from hyperglycemia from several mechanisms including glucose-mediated endothelial damage, oxidative stress, and advanced glycation end products.[8] The incidence of DPN in patients with type 1 and type 2 diabetes mellitus (DM) varies by study, partly based on populations and the way that the neuropathy is diagnosed, but likely is 40% or more with a 10-year history of diabetes. Prediabetes also seems to be a risk factor for the development of DPN (**Table 2** for diagnostic criteria). Multiple studies show a higher prevalence of peripheral neuropathy in those with prediabetes.[9,10]

In some aspects, the amount of nerve injury in those with hyperglycemia seems to be "dose dependent" in that those with longer duration and less well controlled diabetes have a higher incidence of polyneuropathy and more evidence of axonal loss than those with shorter duration and better control. A recent study that followed patients with diabetes and prediabetes found that over 10 years, sural amplitude decreased as hemoglobin A_{1c} increased, and for every 1% increase in hemoglobin

Table 2
Diagnostic criteria for prediabetes and diabetes

Diagnosis	Fasting Plasma Glucose (mg/dL)	HbA$_{1c}$ (%)	2-h Oral Glucose Tolerance Test (mg/dL)
Normal	<100	<5.7	<140
Prediabetes	100–125	5.7–6.4	140–199
Diabetes	>126	>6.5	>200

Data from American Diabetes Association. (2) Classification and diagnosis of diabetes. Diabetes Care 2015;38 Suppl:S8–16.

A_{1C}, sural amplitude diminished by about 1%.[11] Other studies have also noted this primarily axonal destruction as the most common seen in those with altered glucose metabolism.[12]

Beyond Hyperglycemia

However, there is more to the onset and progression of neuropathy in those with metabolic syndrome than just hyperglycemia.[3] One piece of evidence for this is the poor link between improvement in neuropathy rates and blood sugars in those with type 2 DM. In type 1 DM, multiple studies show that enhanced glucose control can substantially reduce the incidence of DPN, and that long-term poor glycemic control is a factor in the rapid development of DPN.[9] In type 2 DM the incidence of polyneuropathy is about the same as those with type 1 DM, but the link between glucose control and neuropathy is not nearly as strong, and intensive glucose control has only a small effect at reducing the incidence of DPN in this population. For example, the ACCORD study followed more than 10,000 patients with DM type 2 and evidence of cardiovascular disease or metabolic syndrome to assess the amount of microvascular damage in those with typical glucose control and those with intensive glucose control (hemoglobin A_{1c} <6) for more than 3 years. Mean time of having DM in this population was 10 years. They used the Michigan Neuropathy Screening index as the diagnostic standard. They found that 45% of those in the usual glucose control had neuropathy, and 43% of those in the intensive glucose control group had neuropathy.[13]

A population-based study of 1256 participants in which the signs and symptoms of neuropathy and nerve conduction studies were performed found a strong association of metabolic syndrome with polyneuropathy whether or not they had diabetes. The more components of the syndrome the participants possessed, the higher the chance of having neuropathy. Central obesity and dyslipidemia particularly were associated with the presence of polyneuropathy.[4,14]

Other factors that may be involved in those with metabolic syndrome and neuropathy are discussed next.

Obesity

The prevalence of polyneuropathy is high in obese patients, even those with normoglycemia. Waist circumference seems to specifically correlate with presence of DPN. For example, in a study of 102 obese patients, 4% in the lean control group had polyneuropathy, 11% in the obese patients with normoglycemia had neuropathy, 30% of those in the obese prediabetes group had neuropathy, and 35% of those in the obese diabetic group had neuropathy.[3] Another study of 908 people in a population-based sample of people without neuropathy symptoms found that participants with increased body mass index had low sural and fibular motor amplitudes on nerve conduction studies. Obesity is also a risk factor for entrapment neuropathies and lumbar radiculopathy.[6,15] This may have a dual mechanism that includes a risk of nerve injury related to metabolic and biomechanical factors.

Dyslipidemia

The link between dyslipidemia and neuropathy is not as clear, but there is some evidence for this connection. There are likely multiple mechanisms involved including oxidative stress, mitochondrial dysregulation, and the role of free fatty acids. Large observational studies have found that those with DM type 2 and abnormal lipid profile go on to develop DPN more than those with normal lipid profiles[16] and at least one study has found a link between elevated triglycerides and the progression of neuropathy, although others have not found these links so the exact link and mechanisms remain unknown.[9]

Hypertension

The link between this aspect of the metabolic syndrome and polyneuropathy remains unclear and based on the literature seems to be the least likely factor in metabolic syndrome to contribute to neuropathy.

TYPES OF NEUROPATHY SEEN IN METABOLIC SYNDROME
Polyneuropathy

The typical polyneuropathy associated with metabolic syndrome is a sensorimotor polyneuropathy that is symmetric and length dependent. Atypical polyneuropathies are also see in metabolic syndrome but are less well studied and beyond the scope of this review.

Clinical diagnosis of polyneuropathy

Symptoms Typical symptoms include foot numbness, paresthesias, or pain. However, symptoms alone are inadequate to make the diagnosis of neuropathy. For example, in a study of 588 patients with type 2 DM where the diagnostic standard was an abnormal clinical neurologic examination, the symptom of daily numbness in the feet had only 22% sensitivity and 92% specificity in patients older than age 68, and 28% sensitivity and 93% specificity in younger patients for presence of neuropathy.[17] The presence of other symptoms, such as pain in the feet, had even worse diagnostic accuracy, and was about the same as chance alone in predicting neuropathy. If patients are evaluated by a battery of questions related to neuropathic symptoms, the sensitivity improves, but specificity is lowered.[18]

Physical examination signs Common physical examination signs in patients with neuropathy include absent Achilles reflexes; impaired great toe proprioception; and decreased sensation, including vibratory, cold, pinprick, and two-point discrimination. Distal weakness is a physical examination finding in severe disease. Isolated physical examination signs, such as absent Achilles reflex or absent proprioception, has high specificity, but lower sensitivity. Composite examination findings of multiple abnormalities have higher diagnostic accuracy than any isolated examination finding.[18]

However, even among neuromuscular experts who were participating in a study to judge diagnostic accuracy, the judgment of physicians about neuropathic signs, symptoms, and diagnosis was excessively variable.[19] It is likely even more so when performed by physicians who are not neuromuscular experts in the context of a busy clinic.

Specialized clinical protocols Likely because of this high variability among clinicians in criteria used and clinical skills necessary to diagnose DPN, a variety of screening protocols have been devised that combine history and physical examination findings to determine the likelihood of neuropathy. One issue with these protocols is that when various screening protocols are used to detect diabetic neuropathy on the same patient, the results are highly variable. For example, in a study in which 142 patients with diabetes underwent three different commonly used clinical screening tests for neuropathy, the authors found poor agreement between the tests. The rate of neuropathy as diagnosed by the screening test in this population varied between nearly 55% for one test and 10% for another.[20] Obesity significantly reduced the reliability of some screening tests.[21]

Asymptomatic polyneuropathy Another factor that argues against the use of signs and symptoms alone to make a diagnosis of DPN is that up to half of patients with diabetes with polyneuropathy are asymptomatic despite extensive physiologic changes and consequences that can lead to muscle atrophy, skin ulcers, bone density changes, and functional deficits, such as unsteadiness and falls.[2,22]

The role of electrodiagnostic studies in diagnosis

Abnormalities of nerve conduction study are the first objective indicator of polyneuropathy. Most experts, such as the Polyneuropathy Task Force, a group of physicians with representatives from the American Academy of Neurology, the American Academy of Physical Medicine and Rehabilitation, and the American Association of Neuromuscular and Electrodiagnostic Medicine, recommend electrodiagnostic testing along with clinical signs and symptoms as the most accurate way to make the diagnosis. Electrodiagnostic studies add a higher level of specificity to the diagnosis than history and physical alone. They also provide a sensitive assessment of the functional status of the nerve that cannot be gathered by other methods. The exact electrodiagnostic criteria to make this diagnosis varies somewhat among experts. In a consensus paper by the Polyneuropathy Task Force, they noted criteria for research purposes, but stated it may be helpful for clinicians. They recommend the minimum criteria of abnormalities of any attribute of nerve conduction in two separate nerves, one of which must be the sural nerve. The suggested protocol is shown in **Fig. 1**. A variety of distal and proximal muscles should be sampled by needle electromyogram if a neuropathy is found. This assists in determining the severity (see later).

Electrodiagnosis to determine causes of neuropathy

In patients referred to a specialist as "idiopathic" neuropathy, most in which a cause is found have either diabetes or prediabetes.[23] Clearly, for these previously undiagnosed patients, electrodiagnostic studies play a key role in uncovering a diagnosis that requires treatment. In addition, electrodiagnostic studies play a pivotal role in the search for causes of polyneuropathy beyond metabolic syndrome, because clearly the diagnosis of metabolic syndrome is not protective of developing other types of treatable neuropathy. By analyzing electrodiagnostic features, other causes that require specific treatment, such as chronic inflammatory demyelinating polyneuropathy, autoimmune diseases, and vitamin deficiencies, may be found. Studies have found that 10% to 50% of patients with diabetes may have an additional cause of their peripheral neuropathy.[5]

Multiple studies have shown the importance of electrodiagnostic studies in diagnosing patients with neuropathic symptoms and how they are used to change patient management.[24] For example, when compared with clinical impression alone, one study found that electrodiagnostic studies confirmed the impression in only 39%, and changed the diagnosis or uncovered additional diagnoses in 43%.[25] Another study found that 37% of patients had a different diagnosis than referring diagnosis.[26] In those with well-established neuropathy risk factors, such as diabetes, electrodiagnostic studies can particularly add value if the presentation is somewhat atypical, such as in the case of asymmetry, weakness, or a subacute or acute onset.[27]

Table 3 provides additional reasons to obtain electrodiagnostic studies in a patient with metabolic syndrome and suspected DPN.

Electrodiagnosis to assess severity of neuropathy

Sensory nerve action potentials to determine severity In typical DPN, sensory nerve action potential abnormalities are the first objective evidence of neuropathy and therefore are sensitive in making the diagnosis. Sensory nerve action potential amplitude is

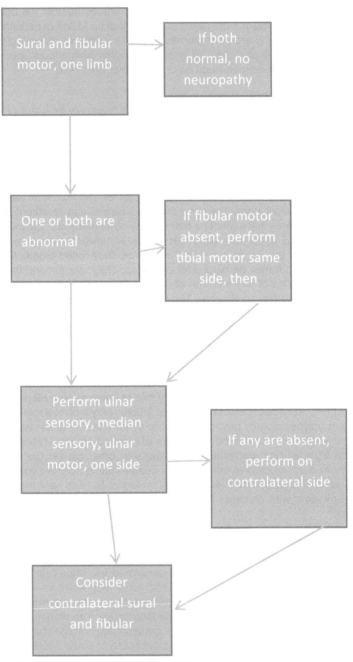

Fig. 1. Simplified nerve conduction studies (NCS) protocol of polyneuropathy task force. (*Data from* England JD, Gronseth GS, Franklin G, et al. Distal symmetrical polyneuropathy: definition for clinical research. Muscle Nerve 2005;31(1):113–23.)

Table 3
Some examples of how electrodiagnostic studies can change patient management in those with metabolic syndrome and suspected polyneuropathy

#	Reason	Example	Type of Intervention
1	Confirm diagnosis	Using signs and symptoms alone can lead to diagnostic errors	Direct treatment to correct cause
2	Uncover additional diagnoses	Carpal tunnel syndrome, radiculopathy	Surgery, injections
3	Diagnose in asymptomatic abnormals	Many patients with peripheral neuropathy present with foot ulcer as first symptom[44]	Foot inspection, proper skin care
4	Identify high-risk patients	Presence of polyneuropathy is associated with greater mortality, increased hospitalizations, and decline in health-related quality of life, among other factors[45]	Population-based medicine to target resources
5	Focus functional interventions	Reduced peripheral nerve function is associated with decreased physical function, such as poor balance, falls, more difficulty arising from a chair, and slowed walking speed.[46]	Physical therapy
6	Correct attribution of neuropathy cause	10%–50% of patients with diabetes may have an additional cause of their peripheral neuropathy[5]	Chronic inflammatory demyelinating polyneuropathy treatment, vitamin B_{12} supplementation, many other
7	Objective data for patient education	Patient self-assessment of foot health is unreliable; in one study of patients with diabetes, nearly 70% of those who considered their feet to be normal had a peripheral neuropathy[44]	Knowledge is essential for behavioral change

a rough indicator of axonal number, particularly in the same patient over time. Because axonal polyneuropathies are length dependent, an abnormality of the medial and lateral planter nerves may assist in diagnosing an early peripheral neuropathy, even if sural is still within the normal range.[28]

Compound motor action potentials to determine severity Amplitude may be preserved if axonal regeneration keeps up with axonal degeneration. In this case, sometimes there is a slight prolongation of distal latency and slightly prolonged conduction velocity because the regenerated axons are thinly myelinated. Low amplitudes therefore suggest a severe polyneuropathy where the healing mechanism of axonal regeneration cannot keep pace with axonal loss.[28]

Needle electromyogram to determine severity This portion of the study is sensitive for detecting even minor axonal loss that may not be appreciated on nerve conduction studies. Positive sharp waves and fibrillation potentials, and other spontaneous activity, such as fasciculations, myokymic discharges, and complex repetitive discharges, may be seen. However, if the disease is progressing slowly, collateral sprouting may keep up with axonal loss and there are not these changes, even in the presence of severe disease. Voluntary motor unit action potentials, however, detect this. There is evidence of terminal reorganization and motor unit remodeling. Appearance varies depending on the stage of the process, and includes increased polyphasicity, duration, and amplitude. A proximal distal gradient is typically found, with the most severe changes in the most distal muscles. Changes should be roughly symmetric. If this is not the pattern seen, competing diagnoses should be considered. Often multiple diagnoses are uncovered, such as the presence of a length-dependent neuropathy with symmetric changes in multiple distal muscles, and a radiculopathy showing changes in a myotome distribution that is asymmetric **(Table 4)**.[28]

For research purposes, composite scores of electrodiagnostic abnormalities are used to classify patients.[29]

Common pitfalls to avoid when performing electrodiagnosis to assess for peripheral neuropathy

Poor technique leading to a "normal" study in patients with neuropathy It is important that electrodiagnostic studies are designed and performed by experts using meticulous standard techniques and appropriately interpreted. In a review of 6381 commercial claims for electrodiagnostic studies in patients with diabetes, the authors found that even when controlling for case mix characteristics, physicians who performed electrodiagnostic studies diagnosed polyneuropathy in six times the number of patients than nonphysician examiners (eg, podiatrist and physical therapist) identified neuropathy (about 12% for physicians vs 2% for nonphysicians.) Given the incidence of polyneuropathy in patients with diabetes, many cases must have been missed.[30]

Table 4
Spectrum of changes seen to determine neuropathy severity

Type of Study	Early/Mild	More Severe	Very Severe
SNAP	Decreased amplitude of longest nerves, such as medial and lateral plantar and sural	More loss of amplitude or absent	Absent
CMAP	Normal or mildly slow distal latency and CV of distal responses	Loss of amplitude, slowed responses, changes seen in more proximal NCS (eg, the hands)	Very low amplitude, slowed distal latency and CV or absent
Needle EMG Spontaneous changes	May be present or not, depending on rate of axonal loss and regeneration	Same as mild	Present as axonal loss overwhelms the ability to regenerate
Needle EMG MUAP	Sensitive for terminal reorganization to make up for axonal loss	More motor units show increased polyphasicity, increased duration, and increased amplitude	Recruitment becomes reduced as axonal loss progresses; remaining motor units show evidence of terminal reorganization

Abbreviations: CMAP, compound motor action potentials; CV, conduction velocity; EMG, electromyogram; MUAP, motor unit action potentials; NCS, nerve conduction studies; SNAP, sensory nerve action potentials.

Data from Dumitru D, Amato AA, Zwarts MJ. Electrodiagnostic medicine. 2nd edition. Philadelphia: Hanley & Belfus; 2002.

In a study of healthy elderly age 60 to 89, a total of 98% had sural nerve responses, and 90% had superficial fibular responses. An absent sural is an abnormal study.[31]

Cool limb leading to "normal" amplitude Inattention to temperature is a common source of error in electrodiagnostic studies. Achieving and maintaining a warm limb for nerve conduction study may be particularly challenging in patients with metabolic syndrome because of the high prevalence of vascular disease, which can lead to cool limbs. If a limb is cool, amplitudes may be interpreted as normal. Using corrective factors rather than warming the limb is typically not adequate, because the effect of cooling on abnormal nerves is not the same as normal nerves.[28]

Poor technique leading to an "abnormal study" in those without neuropathy The incidence of metabolic syndrome increases with aging, so the ability to interpret data in this population is a key skill. The result of aging of a normal nerve causes nerve conduction studies to slow, a drop in the amplitude, prolongation of distal latency, and slowed conduction velocity.[28] Thus, if normative data collected on patients 18 to 24 are used to interpret a study in someone in their 70s, a normal nerve could be classified as abnormal.

Patients with metabolic syndrome are at increased risk of congestive heart failure, renal disease, and vascular disease. These problems can cause lower extremity edema, and skin changes related to chronic edema. This may cause responses to have low amplitude or even be unobtainable. Skin should be carefully prepared for nerve studies, and the amount of edema taken into account when interpreting studies.

Cool limb can lead to misinterpretation of "prolonged distal latency or slowed conduction velocity." Again, limb temperature is a key factor that must be monitored for an accurate study.

Interpreting mild slowing in a tall patient as abnormal Although not fully characterized, tall patients have been shown to have slightly slower distal nerve conduction velocities. This is thought to be secondary to axonal tapering causing smaller fiber diameter at the end of very long limb. Anatomic studies have found slowing of 3.8 m/s for every extra 10 cm of axonal length when comparing distal with proximal responses.[28]

Missing the presence of anomalous innervation Detecting anomalous innervations is challenging in this population because many of the patients are obese. The presence of an accessory fibular nerve is misinterpreted as low fibular motor amplitude if low amplitude is obtained at the ankle, and a submaximal stimulation is performed proximally, which is particularly easy to do if there is a significant overlying adipose. This is then interpreted as adequate stimulation because it "matches" the distal amplitude.

Martin-Gruber anastomoses is similarly missed by submaximal stimulation at the elbow because of overlying adipose, but this typically has less clinical significance because the distal response is not characterized as abnormal as it is in the case of accessory fibular innervation.

Other conditions that cause muscle atrophy masquerading as neuropathy Long-term sequelae from a stroke, which are more common in this population, can lead to foot muscular atrophy. Radiculopathy and spinal stenosis, both of which are more common in this population than healthy control subjects, can cause low-amplitude motor responses. From the authors experience in teaching electrodiagnostic skills, missing the presence of an L5 radiculopathy, particularly a remote radiculopathy that no longer causes symptoms, and instead interpreting this as a fibular neuropathy is particularly common.

Metabolic Syndrome and Radiculopathy

Complex differential diagnosis

Another important reason to perform electrodiagnosis is to rule out competing diagnoses. The study varies depending on patient symptoms, but commonly the competing diagnoses to exclude in a patient with bilateral foot numbness or pain, and physical examination signs, such as decreased sensation and absent Achilles reflexes, is peripheral neuropathy versus spinal stenosis or multiple radiculopathies. Electrodiagnosis is extremely helpful in differentiating between these diagnoses.

Metabolic syndrome as a risk factor

Patients with metabolic syndrome are at increased risk for spine disease. For example, in a study of more than 1500 patients, the presence of all four metabolic syndrome risk factors nearly quadrupled the odds of having severe osteoarthritis of the spine compared with those with no metabolic syndrome risk factors. Obesity has been the best explored risk factor related to metabolic syndrome. Obese patients are at higher risk of low back pain and sciatica.[6] They also have an increased incidence of clinically diagnosed and radiologically diagnosed spinal stenosis. For example, in a Swedish cohort study of more than 350,000 workers who were followed for 39 years, obese subjects had more than twice the risk of developing spinal stenosis compared with those of normal weight.[32]

There is little literature regarding whether other aspects of the metabolic syndrome contribute to radiculopathy. An animal model of radiculopathy in diabetic rats found that they were at increased risk of prolonged neuropathic pain, inflammation, and altered nerve regeneration compared with nondiabetic animals, but this has not been investigated in humans to our knowledge.[33]

People with diabetes are at increased risk of radiculoplexus neuropathy, but it is unknown if other aspects of metabolic syndrome increase the risk of this disease.[34]

Entrapment Neuropathies

Carpal tunnel syndrome: model entrapment

Risk of development Entrapment of the median nerve at the wrist (ie, carpal tunnel syndrome [CTS]) is the most common entrapment neuropathy and the most well studied in metabolic syndrome. In a case series of patients diagnose with CTS, 75% of patients with CTS were found to have metabolic syndrome. The electrophysiologic parameters were also more abnormal in those with metabolic syndrome than those without.[35]

Several components of the metabolic syndrome seem to be particularly associated with CTS. Excess body mass seems to be an especially strong risk factor. In a metanalysis of 58 studies involving more than 1.3 million subjects, they found a dose-dependent link between weight and CTS in those overweight and obese. Each one unit increase in body mass index increased the risk of CTS by more than 7.4%. Being obese increased the risk two-fold over normal-weight subjects.[36] As in some other medical conditions, increased waist circumference and high waist to hip ratio seems to be particularly harmful.[15]

Prediabetes is another risk factor for CTS, one that is often undiagnosed in this setting. For example, in an Italian study of 117 patients with chronic idiopathic CTS, 45% had an abnormal 2-hour glucose tolerance test, and an additional 14% had undiagnosed diabetes. The increased incidence of impaired glucose metabolism in those with CTS remained significant even when controlled for waist circumference and obesity, so it seems to be an independent risk factor within the metabolic syndrome, and the authors suggested all patients with idiopathic CTS should undergo glucose tolerance testing.[37] Diabetes is also a well-known risk factor for CTS. Entrapment neuropathies may go undiagnosed in patients with diabetes because their symptoms may be attributed to length-dependent polyneuropathy rather than a treatable entrapment.

Treatment and outcomes in those with metabolic syndrome Despite their comorbidities, these patients can respond to treatment of their CTS. At least one study has shown that patients with hypertension, obesity, or statin treatment had a similar improvement after carpal tunnel release surgery than patients without these diagnoses.[7]

The outcome of carpal tunnel release in patients with diabetes has also been analyzed. Although patients with DM and CTS typically have more impaired neurophysiologic findings than those without diabetes and CTS, researchers found that from baseline to 1 year and from 1 year to 5 years, patients with diabetes and without diabetes had significant improvement in neurophysiologic findings and even those patients with peripheral neuropathy had improvement. However, when adjusted for baseline differences in nerve conduction study values, diabetes did have a negative impact on neurophysiologic improvement. This is consistent with studies that show improvement of clinical symptoms in patients with diabetes who have had carpal tunnel release, although some studies have shown the improvement is not as robust as those without diabetes.[38,39]

Other entrapments

Ulnar neuropathy at the elbow is the second most common entrapment neuropathy, and also has an increased incidence in patients with diabetes. Because of the pathology seen in nerves in patients with metabolic syndrome, entrapments in the lower limb may be more likely than in the general population, but they have not been as well studied.[40]

Role of electrodiagnosis in diagnosing entrapment neuropathies

Electrodiagnosis plays a key role in diagnosing entrapment neuropathies in all patients and is even more essential in those with metabolic syndrome because of the high incidence of disorders in the differential diagnoses of entrapment neuropathies. For example, many symptoms of hand osteoarthritis and CTS overlap. Patients with metabolic syndrome, particularly obese patients, have an increased risk of hand osteoarthritis. For example, a large population study found obesity was significantly associated with hand osteoarthritis with an odds ratio of 2.59.[41] Other features of the metabolic syndrome, hypertension, and type 2 diabetes have been found to be independent risk factors from obesity in the development of osteoarthritis. This is likely caused by chronic, low-level inflammation associated with metabolic syndrome.[42] Given the high incidence of CTS and hand arthritis in this population, it is likely that symptomatic patients may have both conditions, and both need to be diagnosed for proper treatment.

Electrodiagnosis in those with metabolic syndrome and possible entrapment neuropathies: common pitfalls

Challenges in the obese patient It may be particularly challenging to diagnose ulnar neuropathy at the elbow (ie, cubital tunnel syndrome) and fibular neuropathy at the fibular head in obese patients. Ideally, entrapment neuropathies are diagnosed by stimulating the nerve below and above the area of entrapment and analyzing whether there is slowing of nerve conduction, and/or presence of conduction block revealed by a loss of amplitude in the proximal response. In obese patients this is technically challenging. Surface measurements of distance between stimulation points, which is necessary to calculate conduction velocity, may be inaccurate because of the presence of adipose tissue. In addition, because the nerve is further from the stimulation site if there is overlying adipose tissue, it may be difficult to achieve enough electrical stimulation to obtain accurate amplitude in the more proximal stimulation sites, leading to a misdiagnosis of conduction block. Sometimes, this pitfall is avoided by doing side-to-side comparison studies, but if symptoms are bilateral, this is not as helpful.

Diagnosing entrapment in presence of polyneuropathy In a patient with length-dependent polyneuropathy, hand symptoms warrant a search for treatable entrapments with an electrodiagnostic evaluation because of the high incidence of entrapments in this population and the difficulty of sorting out entrapments by signs and symptoms in a patient who also has neuropathy.

Sufficient comparison studies must be done to ensure that the abnormalities seen in nerve conduction studies are from local entrapment and not a diffuse peripheral neuropathy. Evaluating only the nerve that is symptomatic and diagnosing an entrapment is not sufficient in patients with metabolic syndrome. Such techniques as combined sensory index to evaluate for the presence of slowing within the carpal tunnel add sufficient sensitivity and specificity to make this diagnosis even in the presence of peripheral neuropathy.[43] This principle of evaluating other nerves in the vicinity is applied to other entrapments. For example, when evaluating for injury of the fibular nerve at the fibular head in someone with metabolic syndrome, it is important to test both the sural and superficial fibular nerve to evaluate for the presence of a sensory neuropathy, and the tibial or contralateral fibular nerve to assess for a more widespread polyneuropathy.

Diagnosing polyneuropathy in the presence of entrapment Some experts recommend that a search for a length-dependent polyneuropathy is essential for patients with metabolic syndrome and an entrapment neuropathy because of the high incidence of these disorders occurring together and the high risk of missing a length-dependent polyneuropathy. Often prediabetes and even diabetes may go undiagnosed in this population, and an entrapment neuropathy could be the presenting symptom.[37]

SUMMARY

Metabolic syndrome is an increasing common disorder. Patients with metabolic syndrome are at increased risk of multiple peripheral nerve problems, even in those with normal glucose metabolism. Diagnosis of nerve disease in this population is challenging. Differential diagnosis of symptoms may be broad because of metabolic syndrome's impact on many diseases. A carefully designed and performed electrodiagnostic evaluation can add valuable information that changes patient care. Besides leading to a correct diagnosis, and often uncovering more than one diagnosis, electrodiagnosis adds value in other ways, such as determining the severity of nerve damage, identifying patients at high risk for functional problems, and providing valuable information to patients about their health.

REFERENCES

1. Aguilar M, Bhuket T, Torres S, et al. Prevalence of the metabolic syndrome in the United States, 2003-2012. JAMA 2015;313(19):1973–4.

2. Pop-Busui R, Boulton AJ, Feldman EL, et al. Diabetic neuropathy: a position statement by the American Diabetes Association. Diabetes Care 2017;40(1):136–54.

3. Callaghan BC, Xia R, Reynolds E, et al. Association between metabolic syndrome components and polyneuropathy in an obese population. JAMA Neurol 2016;73(12):1468–76.

4. Hanewinckel R, Drenthen J, Ligthart S, et al. Metabolic syndrome is related to polyneuropathy and impaired peripheral nerve function: a prospective population-based cohort study. J Neurol Neurosurg Psychiatry 2016;87(12):1336–42.

5. Freeman R. Not all neuropathy in diabetes is of diabetic etiology: differential diagnosis of diabetic neuropathy. Curr Diab Rep 2009;9(6):423–31.

6. Shiri R, Lallukka T, Karppinen J, et al. Obesity as a risk factor for sciatica: a meta-analysis. Am J Epidemiol 2014;179(8):929–37.

7. Zimmerman M, Dahlin E, Thomsen NOB, et al. Outcome after carpal tunnel release: impact of factors related to metabolic syndrome. J Plast Surg Hand Surg 2017;51(3):165–71.

8. Khalil H. Diabetes microvascular complications: a clinical update. Diabetes Metab Syndr 2017;11(Suppl 1):S133–9.

9. Grisold A, Callaghan BC, Feldman EL. Mediators of diabetic neuropathy: is hyperglycemia the only culprit? Curr Opin Endocrinol Diabetes Obes 2017;24(2):103–11.

10. Singleton JR, Smith AG, Bromberg MB. Increased prevalence of impaired glucose tolerance in patients with painful sensory neuropathy. Diabetes Care 2001;24(8):1448–53.

11. Peterson M, Pingel R, Lagali N, et al. Association between HbA1c and peripheral neuropathy in a 10-year follow-up study of people with normal glucose tolerance, impaired glucose tolerance and type 2 diabetes. Diabet Med 2017;34(12):1756–64.

12. Partanen J, Niskanen L, Lehtinen J, et al. Natural history of peripheral neuropathy in patients with non-insulin-dependent diabetes mellitus. N Engl J Med 1995;333(2):89–94.

13. Ismail-Beigi F, Craven T, Banerji MA, et al. Effect of intensive treatment of hyperglycaemia on microvascular outcomes in type 2 diabetes: an analysis of the ACCORD randomised trial. Lancet 2010;376(9739):419–30.

14. Hanewinckel R, Ikram MA, Franco OH, et al. High body mass and kidney dysfunction relate to worse nerve function, even in adults without neuropathy. J Peripher Nerv Syst 2017;22(2):112–20.

15. Mondelli M, Aretini A, Ginanneschi F, et al. Waist circumference and waist-to-hip ratio in carpal tunnel syndrome: a case-control study. J Neurol Sci 2014;338(1–2):207–13.

16. Perez-Matos MC, Morales-Alvarez MC, Mendivil CO. Lipids: a suitable therapeutic target in diabetic neuropathy? J Diabetes Res 2017;2017:6943851.

17. Franse LV, Di Bari M, Shorr RI, et al. Type 2 diabetes in older well-functioning people: who is undiagnosed? Data from the health, aging, and body composition study. Diabetes Care 2001;24(12):2065–70.

18. England JD, Gronseth GS, Franklin G, et al. Distal symmetrical polyneuropathy: definition for clinical research. Muscle Nerve 2005;31(1):113–23.

19. Dyck PJ, Overland CJ, Low PA, et al. Signs and symptoms versus nerve conduction studies to diagnose diabetic sensorimotor polyneuropathy: CI vs. NPhys trial. Muscle Nerve 2010;42(2):157–64.

20. Forouzandeh F, Aziz Ahari A, Abolhasani F, et al. Comparison of different screening tests for detecting diabetic foot neuropathy. Acta Neurol Scand 2005;112(6):409–13.

21. Boyraz O, Saracoglu M. The effect of obesity on the assessment of diabetic peripheral neuropathy: a comparison of Michigan patient version test and Michigan physical assessment. Diabetes Res Clin Pract 2010;90(3):256–60.

22. Hanewinckel R, Drenthen J, Verlinden VJA, et al. Polyneuropathy relates to impairment in daily activities, worse gait, and fall-related injuries. Neurology 2017;89(1):76–83.

23. Farhad K, Traub R, Ruzhansky KM, et al. Causes of neuropathy in patients referred as "idiopathic neuropathy". Muscle Nerve 2016;53(6):856–61.

24. Bodofsky EB, Carter GT, England JD. Is electrodiagnostic testing for polyneuropathy overutilized? Muscle Nerve 2017;55(3):301–4.

25. Cho SC, Siao-Tick-Chong P, So YT. Clinical utility of electrodiagnostic consultation in suspected polyneuropathy. Muscle Nerve 2004;30(5):659–62.

26. Kothari MJ, Blakeslee MA, Reichwein R, et al. Electrodiagnostic studies: are they useful in clinical practice? Arch Phys Med Rehabil 1998;79(12):1510–1.

27. Callaghan BC, Burke JF, Kerber KA, et al. Electrodiagnostic tests are unlikely to change management in those with a known cause of typical distal symmetric polyneuropathy. Muscle Nerve 2017;56(3):E25.

28. Dumitru D, Amato AA, Zwarts MJ. Electrodiagnostic medicine. 2nd edition. Philadelphia: Hanley & Belfus; 2002.

29. Dyck PJ, Albers JW, Andersen H, et al. Diabetic polyneuropathies: update on research definition, diagnostic criteria and estimation of severity. Diabetes Metab Res Rev 2011;27(7):620–8.

30. Dillingham TR, Pezzin LE. Under-recognition of polyneuropathy in persons with diabetes by nonphysician electrodiagnostic services providers. Am J Phys Med Rehabil 2005;84(6):399–406.

31. Falco FJ, Hennessey WJ, Goldberg G, et al. Standardized nerve conduction studies in the lower limb of the healthy elderly. Am J Phys Med Rehabil 1994;73(3):168–74.

32. Knutsson B, Sanden B, Sjoden G, et al. Body mass index and risk for clinical lumbar spinal stenosis: a cohort study. Spine (Phila Pa 1976) 2015;40(18):1451–6.

33. Kameda T, Sekiguchi M, Kaneuchi Y, et al. Investigation of the effect of diabetes on radiculopathy induced by nucleus pulposus application to the DRG in a spontaneously diabetic rat model. Spine (Phila Pa 1976) 2017;42(23):1749–56.

34. Massie R, Mauermann ML, Staff NP, et al. Diabetic cervical radiculoplexus neuropathy: a distinct syndrome expanding the spectrum of diabetic radiculoplexus neuropathies. Brain 2012;135(Pt 10):3074–88.

35. Balci K, Utku U. Carpal tunnel syndrome and metabolic syndrome. Acta Neurol Scand 2007;116(2):113–7.

36. Shiri R, Pourmemari MH, Falah-Hassani K, et al. The effect of excess body mass on the risk of carpal tunnel syndrome: a meta-analysis of 58 studies. Obes Rev 2015;16(12):1094–104.

37. Plastino M, Fava A, Carmela C, et al. Insulin resistance increases risk of carpal tunnel syndrome: a case-control study. J Peripher Nerv Syst 2011;16(3):186–90.

38. Thomsen NOB, Andersson GS, Bjork J, et al. Neurophysiological recovery 5 years after carpal tunnel release in patients with diabetes. Muscle Nerve 2017;56(6):E59–64.

39. Gulabi D, Cecen G, Guclu B, et al. Carpal tunnel release in patients with diabetes result in poorer outcome in long-term study. Eur J Orthop Surg Traumatol 2014; 24(7):1181–4.

40. Rota E, Morelli N. Entrapment neuropathies in diabetes mellitus. World J Diabetes 2016;7(17):342–53.

41. Grotle M, Hagen KB, Natvig B, et al. Obesity and osteoarthritis in knee, hip and/or hand: an epidemiological study in the general population with 10 years follow-up. BMC Musculoskelet Disord 2008;9:132.

42. Sellam J, Berenbaum F. Is osteoarthritis a metabolic disease? Joint Bone Spine 2013;80(6):568–73.

43. Robinson LR. Electrodiagnosis of carpal tunnel syndrome. Phys Med Rehabil Clin N Am 2007;18(4):733–46, vi.

44. Baba M, Duff J, Foley L, et al. A comparison of two methods of foot health education: the Fremantle Diabetes Study Phase II. Prim Care Diabetes 2015;9(2): 155–62.

45. Mold JW, Lawler F, Roberts M, Oklahoma Physicians Resource/Research Network Study. The health consequences of peripheral neurological deficits in an elderly cohort: an Oklahoma Physicians Resource/Research Network Study. J Am Geriatr Soc 2008;56(7):1259–64.

46. Strotmeyer ES, de Rekeneire N, Schwartz AV, et al. The relationship of reduced peripheral nerve function and diabetes with physical performance in older white and black adults: the Health, Aging, and Body Composition (Health ABC) study. Diabetes Care 2008;31(9):1767–72.

Guiding Treatment for Carpal Tunnel Syndrome

Leilei Wang, MD, PhD

KEYWORDS

- Carpal tunnel syndrome • Neuropathy • Nerve conduction studies
- Electrodiagnosis

KEY POINTS

- Making the correct carpal tunnel syndrome diagnosis is the most important step in treatment. Electrodiagnosis can confirm carpal tunnel syndrome and eliminate mimicking diseases from the differential.
- Treatment should provide satisfactory pain relief and protection of the median nerve from further deterioration.
- The importance and value of reversing focal median mononeuropathy at the wrist in the long term have not been sufficiently addressed, despite its high prevalence and chronic nature.
- Only electrodiagnosis provides information on focal median mononeuropathy at the wrist that could be used to classify carpal tunnel syndrome from mild to severe.
- False positives can cause more harm than false negatives in the case of carpal tunnel syndrome.

INTRODUCTION

Carpal tunnel syndrome (CTS) has long been accepted to be a symptomatic condition caused by compression of the median nerve at the wrist. Historically, the realization that CTS is a clear clinical entity resulting from 1 nerve affected at 1 specific anatomic location took time.[1] Medical understanding of CTS as a focal median mononeuropathy at the wrist (FMMNW) was well-established by the mid-20th century.[2,3] Surgeons treating traumatically injured upper limbs were early pioneers of this field.[4]

Known as the most common focal entrapment mononeuropathy, CTS represents 90% of all entrapment neuropathy and affects millions of Americans. One in 5 ambulatory clinic visits are for CTS, with a reported high incidence and prevalence not only in the United States but in other countries as well. The lifetime risk is estimated to be 10%.[5–8] Both clinicians of general practice and neuromusculoskeletal specialties see,

Disclosure: None.
Department of Rehabilitation Medicine, School of Medicine, University of Washington, 1959 Northeast Pacific Street, Box 356157, Seattle, WA 98195, USA
E-mail address: lw7@uw.edu

diagnose, and treat patients with CTS by recognizing its constellation symptoms and signs and using provocative test, electrodiagnosis (EDX) and more recently imaging modality including computer tomography, magnetic resonance neurography and ultrasound examination.[9–14]

EDX for the diagnosis of CTS has had much in-depth investigation and collective knowledge accumulated since the 1950s.[15] It is especially helpful when the clinical presentation is less straightforward.[16,17] Diagnostic validity has been extensively studied with continuous research interest for further improvements, including the recently published article addressing diagnostic normal values that entailed group consensus and an extensive review of the literature.[18]

Because CTS is such a common and often chronic disease, it has provided physicians and researchers ample opportunities for refining medical treatments and sharing cumulative experiences. There is an impressive volume of literature that is still growing with technological advancements and ongoing academic research. The treatment of CTS, which is typically splinting, corticosteroid injection, and surgery, have been mostly effective.[19,20] Published practice guidelines for treating CTS including the recent guideline by the American Academy of Orthopedic Surgeons, which are endorsed by medical professional organizations including the Academy of Physical Medicine and Rehabilitation and the American Association of Neuromuscular & Electrodiagnostic Medicine.[21]

However, there remain plenty of variations of management with room for discussion and improvement.[22–24] The goal of this article is to review the current literature on the diagnosis and management of CTS, with an emphasis on the role of EDX when treating CTS.

ANATOMY OF THE CARPAL TUNNEL AND MEDIAN NERVE

To understand current CTS treatment practice, a review of median nerve and carpal tunnel anatomy is important. The carpal tunnel is a shallow, U-shaped, bony trough formed by the carpal bones, with the transverse carpal ligament enclosing the open volar side. The carpal tunnel is an inelastic and narrow passage for the median nerve and 9 flexor tendons to travel from the forearm to the hand. The slightly dumbbell-shaped carpal tunnel has a width of 20 to 25 mm. The segment of median nerve traveling inside the carpal tunnel between the levels of the distal wrist flexion crease and the proximal metaphysis is at high risk of becoming entrapped and injured.[25–27]

The median nerve is formed by fascicles from the medial and lateral cord of the brachial plexus. After reaching the elbow, the median nerve sends motor axons to innervate several muscles: the pronator teres, flexor carpi radialis, palmaris longus, and flexor digitorum superficialis. Then, the anterior interosseous nerve branches off, which innervates the flexor digitorum profundus I and II, the flexor pollicis longus and the pronator quadratus muscles. There are several known sites in the arm and forearm that could entrap the median nerve, but these occur with a much lower frequency than at the carpal tunnel. The palmar cutaneous branch of the median nerve piercing through the fascia provides skin sensation of the proximal palm. The remaining median nerve fascicles reach the wrist between the tendons of flexor carpi radialis and palmaris longus and enter the carpal tunnel.

The terminal branches of the median nerve have several proper digital sensory nerves and 1 motor nerve. The proper digital nerves provide sensation to the palmar skin of the thumb, index, and the long and radial sides of the ring fingers, plus the dorsal skin of the distal phalanx of these digits. The terminal motor branch was named the recurrent or thenar nerve because it makes a turnaround in the palm before arriving at the thenar eminence and innervating the abductor pollicis brevis, opponents pollicis, superficial head of the flexor pollicis brevis muscles.

CTS develops when the median nerve is compressed and clinical symptoms occur in the distribution of the anatomy of these terminal branches. Clinical complaints and physical findings in the median nerve distribution are the foundation when diagnosing CTS. However, many sensory and motor anomalies exist. It is beyond the scope of this article, but a keen awareness of these anomalies is important not only to CTS surgery performing carpal tunnel release (CTR) but also to the diagnosis of CTS.[28–30]

CAUSES AND DIAGNOSIS OF CARPAL TUNNEL SYNDROME

Consensus on the cause of the most common idiopathic CTS has been compression and ischemic insult to the short segment of median nerve inside the carpal tunnel. Normal carpal tunnel pressure is less than 5 mm Hg with the wrist in neutral position. Pressure increases with activity and prolonged flexion and extension. For example, it increases to 20 to 30 mm Hg with the use of a computer mouse. Impaired median nerve blood flow occurs at the pressure of 20 to 30 mm Hg. When the median nerve is stressed beyond its physiologic tolerance, CTS symptoms develop.[31,32] Nerves do not like compression or ischemia. With high enough pressure, long enough duration, and associated ischemia, the median nerve begins to develop pathology. The result is FMMNW with sensory demyelination being first, followed by motor demyelination, and eventually sensory and motor axon loss. Risk factors include high body mass index, female gender, age, pregnancy, and many others.[33–35] Stretching and tethering by the surrounding connective tissue like thickened or swollen synovia or bony irregularity are other plausible causes of compression that results in ischemic injury.

Although CTS can resolve spontaneously, it is common for patients diagnosed with CTS to recall similar symptoms in the past with either a gradual worsening or a relapsing–remitting pattern over months, years, or even decades. The most frequent complaints are nighttime burning and "pins-and-needles" pain in the fingers. Acroparaesthesiae is used to describe these sensations.[3] As CTS progresses, pain and numbness is typically felt during the day intermittently, triggered by activities like driving, lifting, or computer use. In many patients, the pain eventually becomes constant. Patients report feeling of swollen hand, clumsiness, and object dropping. Weakness is a late sign associated with thenar atrophy.

Less typical sensory symptoms are frequently reported by many patients, which range from symptoms involving all the fingers, entire hand, forearm, arm, and shoulder. Nonmedian nerve distribution neurologic symptoms alone should not deter one away from CTS suspicion.[36,37]

Pain is a prominent feature of CTS and may limit sensation and strength examination. Adding visual inspection, noting subtle differences when comparing the affected hand with the asymptomatic hand (taking hand dominance into consideration) can be helpful to determine if strength limitations are related to pain or muscle loss.

Many provocative special tests are available.[10,11,38] Besides the classic Tinel and Phalen test, there are many others described in the literature.[39,40] Most are designed to apply stress to the median nerve at the wrist in an attempt to provoke CTS symptoms. These tests could be performed quickly in an ambulatory clinic. The reported sensitivity and specificity of these maneuvers has been variable.[41] Fortunately, when used consistently, and coupled with relevant clinical history and physical examination that includes searching for both the pertinent positive and the pertinent negative information, a diagnosis of CTS can be achieved with reasonable certainty in many CTS cases.

Magnetic resonance neurography and ultrasound imagining can provide additional information such as synovitis and anatomic anomaly.[42,43] In contrast, computed tomography—despite its strength in viewing bones—was reported to have little value.[44]

EDX has been called "the gold standard," when in reality a gold standard does not exist in diagnosing CTS. The use of EDX for CTS has some shortcomings, including a relatively low sensitivity, causing patient discomfort, and the potential of increasing costs. However, many treating physicians and patients appreciate the extra information it provides regarding the diagnosis when making decision on treatment, and also for prognosis.[45] In contrast, imaging studies provide, for the most part, binary data: differentiating a normal versus abnormal appearing median nerve, whereas EDX further provides quantifiable information on the pathology of FMMNW. Although EDX is not necessary to diagnose CTS, its use for confirmation and eliminating other causes are valuable.

Diagnosing CTS becomes more challenging in a patient with diabetes, neck or shoulder pain extending to hand, or traumatic upper limb injuries. EDX is helpful in the diagnosis of peripheral polyneuropathy, cervical radiculopathy, plexopathy, and proximal median mononeuropathy, which can all cause symptoms similar to CTS.

TREATMENT, OUTCOME, AND USEFULNESS OF ELECTRODIAGNOSIS

Treatments are typically grouped into conservative treatments versus surgical treatments. The 2 approaches that have resulted in the most consistent satisfaction are steroid injection and CTR.[5,9] Available treatment outcome research favor steroid injection and surgery.[46,47] Splints used as adjunct treatment seem to improve pain in many patients despite having no significant statistical evidence by Cochrane analysis.[48] Besides pain reduction and sleep improvement, splint use helps some patients to become more ergonomically aware of their hand use while deciding on the treatment based on their individual needs or waiting to be seen by a hand specialist. Some patients afflicted by CTS prefer to delay surgery or avoid it all together. The newest treatment, hydrodissection or transverse carpal ligament release under ultrasound guidance by nonsurgical physicians, is showing promise with research evidence yet to come.[49]

Studies have shown that there seems to be a window for optimal treatment outcomes. Conservative treatments are less effective in reducing CTS symptoms when used for advanced moderate or severe cases. Surgical outcomes are also better in resolving CTS symptoms and the underlying FMMNW when performed for the mild or early moderate CTS.

Has EDX added usefulness in guiding CTS treatment? The author would be the first to point out the potential biases from a skewed viewpoint. Yet, with more than 500 CTS study cases annually in a teaching University EDX laboratory, clinic-based observations could offer some insights. See **Table 1** for examples of how EDX adds value to clinical care.

CTS and FMMNW are often used as synonyms; however, there are some differences, because a syndrome is about symptoms, whereas EDX-positive CTS is more specifically for FMMNW. Trying to predict the severity of FMMNW using CTS symptoms can be misleading. Abnormal EDX findings do not always parallel the severity of CTS symptoms. There are patients with classic CTS symptoms but normal EDX. Abnormal EDX findings are also found in asymptomatic population.[50] The disparity between symptoms and electrodiagnostic findings can even be seen within the same patient when bilateral studies are performed. Surgery, referred to as the

Table 1
Ways that EDX adds value in the diagnosis and treatment of CTS

Reason	Example of Situation	Example of Change in Management
Confirm/refute suspected diagnosis	Patient with hand pain at night	Negative EDX may lead to diagnosis of hand OA or tendinopathy as cause of symptoms
Lead to additional diagnoses	Patient with hand numbness is found to have polyneuropathy with or without CTS	Search for causes of polyneuropathy could lead to diagnosis of Diabetes, Vitamin deficiency, etc.
Find other causes of symptoms	Patient with hand numbness found to have cervical radiculopathy	Treatment of radiculopathy
Pre-CTR data compared with post-CTR data	Patient has recurrent symptoms after CTR	EDX confirms worsening FMMNW and patient treated appropriately OR EDX finds improvement in FMMNW and another etiology sought
Guide treatment	Patient has evidence of worsening FMMNW	Physician does not continue conservative treatment with night splints, but moves to surgical referral
Prognosis	Electrodiagnostic category used to inform discussion about prognosis with surgery	Patient makes informed decision about whether to move forward with elective surgery
Research	EDX confirms diagnosis ("gold standard")	Patients appropriately categorized for study and follow-up

Abbreviations: CTR, carpal tunnel release; CTS, carpal tunnel syndrome; EDX, electrodiagnosis; FMMNW, focal median mononeuropathy at the wrist; OA, osteoarthritis.

"definitive treatment" for CTS, has been shown to relieve CTS symptoms ranging from the EDX-negative group to the group with no recordable median nerve signal.[45,51] Therefore, if the goal is only to cure the symptoms, in cases where the diagnosis is certain, EDX may be unnecessary.

In contrast, EDX adds values in several ways. There is evidence that EDX can be used in predicting outcomes for both the steroid injection and CTR.[52–56] It is also helpful in differentiating mimicking diseases like overuse tendonitis, cervical radiculopathy, peripheral neuropathy, and misleading indicators in cases of trauma.

Having had a pre-CTR EDX study can be helpful when studying the post-CTR symptomatic group. Abnormalities of EDX study improve after CTR. Pre-CTR electrodiagnostic studies are helpful for comparison; even with complete resolution of CTS symptoms, residual EDX abnormality often persist, unless the study result was normal or only mild abnormal before surgery. Post-CTR median motor latencies often return to normal, but the sensory latencies often do not. Absent sensory response on pretesting may return, but the amplitude is often small. The underlying reasons for residual sensory abnormality are not clear but could be because the sensory nerves typically have worse demyelination than motor fibers, and therefore sensory nerve remyelination is less efficient after release. Sensory axon loss could be another mechanism resulting in the residual abnormality given large and fast conducting nerve fibers are more vulnerable to compression and ischemia.

It is important to point out that although current CTS classification schemes differ in details, they all use EDX findings of FMMNW. Researchers use EDX as a tool or an assay to compare pretreatment and posttreatment conditions of CTS.

LOOKING INTO THE FUTURE
Continued Attention to Sensitivity in Making the Diagnosis

The low sensitivity of EDX should be addressed by using the best-published normal values for diagnosis as recommended by the American Association of Neuromuscular & Electrodiagnostic Medicine and using diagnostic criteria less influenced by intrinsic or extrinsic variations. Comparative values are preferred when available over the use of absolute population normal values for making the diagnosis. This is because mild abnormalities can be detected with less influences and potential errors introduced by temperature and other factors. Findings are also more reproducible with interexaminer studies.

Attention to Sensory Amplitudes, Not Just Latency

There are patients who seem to have early median sensory axon loss in addition to sensory demyelination, showing decreased or even absent sensory amplitude while median motor results are well within the normal range. Closer attention to sensory amplitude in addition to sensory latency may be useful in better stratifying CTS for prognosis and outcome research.

Inching and Other Techniques

Short distance nerve conduction studies have been used to measure entrapment neuropathy. This test is used most frequently in the upper limb for the evaluation of ulnar neuropathy at the elbow. There are a few publications on applying inching and other techniques for the study of CTS.[57–59] This test should be revisited and standardized. The author has found it to be valuable in determining the location of median neuropathy in patients with a history of forearm injury in search of treatable CTS.[60]

Clinical Skills and Sound Medical and Technical Knowledge of Electrodiagnosis over Templates and Inflexible Protocols

Clinical skills guide the electrodiagnosticians to choose properly among many established study options and increase the validity when interpreting findings for the individual patient.

Decreasing Patient Discomfort

The associated discomfort of EDX should be decreased. Skilled examining physicians take their time to explain the query (the why) and the study approach (the what) while answering questions and providing the education to the patient that he or she needs. Discomfort extent reported by the patient differs greatly with needle examination generally being the worst, followed by motor conduction study with sensory conduction study being the least bothersome. However, not infrequently, the patient being tested falls asleep during the study in our laboratory. Attention to each patient's individual and unique concerns is important. In addition to using good EDX techniques, making clear to patients that they can stop their study at any time could be valuable while using reassuring and understanding mannerisms. In the author's experience, essentially no one declines to begin the study, and only a few per year opted to stop. Most of these patients rescheduled and completed the study at the second appointment. Conveying knowledge and respect to variable individual tolerance lightens patient's anxiety and worries of "being weak" or even feeling of shame. Many patients are surprised at the ease of the study, with some lamenting their unnecessarily lost sleep the night before from reading information about EDX on the Internet. Pain, fear, and coping capacity with a stressful condition vary greatly from person to person depending on the individual's biology, personality, past experiences, and many other factors. Diagnosing and treating CTS can serve as a reminder for professionals to do the best for each patient and to add no harm.

Better Carpal Tunnel Syndrome Outcome Research

Conducting outcome and outcome comparison studies are time consuming and manpower expensive. Numerous variations, including biology, milieu, experience, and style in seeking medical advice are difficult to control fully. Treating clinicians are likely, often unintentionally, to introduce bias depending on professional training and practice. Currently, most long-term prospective outcome research followed CTS and treatments evaluate this over a few months to a couple of years at most. Outcome studies for a longer period of time will likely be important, not only for choosing treatment options but also from a public health management standpoint given the lifelong risk and the chronic nature of CTS.

Better Prevention and Early Management

Physicians should consider managing CTS similarly to other epidemic and chronic diseases by using education and routine quick checks at regular health visits. With a decrease in the individual's risk of developing CTS and early diagnosis using EDX as indicated, the disease burden of CTS and its associated high medical treatment cost, personal life quality, or work productivity loss could be decreased.[61,62]

REFERENCES

1. Amadio PC. History of carpal tunnel syndrome [Chapter 1]. In: Luchetti R, Amadio PC, editors. Carpal tunnel syndrome. Berlin: Springer; 2007. p. 3–9.
2. Brain WR, Wright AD, Wilkinson M. Spontaneous compression of both median nerves in the carpal tunnel; six cases treated surgically. Lancet 1947;1:277–82.
3. Kremer M, Gilliatt RW, Golding JSB, et al. Acroparaesthesiae in the carpal tunnel-syndrome. Lancet 1953;2:590–5.
4. Phalen GS. The birth of a syndrome, or carpal tunnel revisited. J Hand Surg Am 1981;6:109–10.
5. Ashworth NL. Carpal Tunnel Syndrome. Available at: http://www.emedicine.com/pmr/topic21.htm. Accessed January 2, 2018.
6. Mondelli M, Giannni F, Giacchi M. Carpal tunnel syndrome incidence in a general population. Neurology 2002;58:289–94.
7. Atroshi I, Gummesson C, Johnsson R, et al. Prevalence of carpal tunnel syndrome in a general population. JAMA 1999;282:153–8.
8. Stevens JC, Sun S, Beard CM, et al. Carpal tunnel syndrome in Rochester, Minnesota, 1961–1980. Neurology 1988;38:134–8.
9. Padua L, Coraci D, Erra C, et al. Diagnosis and treatment of carpal tunnel syndrome: clinical features, diagnosis, and management. Lancet Neurol 2016; 15(12):1273–84.
10. MacDermid JC, Wessel J. Clinical diagnosis of carpal tunnel syndrome: a systematic review. J Hand Ther 2004;17(2):309–19.

11. El Miedany Y, Ashour S, Youssef S, et al. Clinical diagnosis of carpal tunnel syndrome: old tests-new concepts. Joint Bone Spine 2008;75:451–7.

12. Werner RA, Andary M. Electrodiagnostic evaluation of carpal tunnel syndrome. Muscle Nerve 2011;44:597–607.

13. Jarvik JG, Yuen E, Haynor DR, et al. MR nerve imaging in a prospective cohort of patients with suspected carpal tunnel syndrome. Neurology 2002;58:1597–602.

14. Kotevoglu N, Gülbahce-Saglam S. Ultrasound imaging in the diagnosis of carpal tunnel syndrome and its relevance to clinical evaluation. Joint Bone Spine 2005; 72:142–5.

15. Simpson JA. Electrical signs in the diagnosis of carpal tunnel and related syndrome. J Neurol Neurosurg Psychiatry 1956;19:275–80.

16. Wang L. Electrodiagnosis of carpal tunnel syndrome. Phys Med Rehabil Clin N Am 2013;24:67–77.

17. Jablecki CK, Andary MT, So YT, et al. Literature review of the usefulness of nerve conduction studies and electromyography in the evaluation of patients with carpal tunnel syndrome. Muscle Nerve 1993;16:1392–414.

18. Chen S, Andary M, Buschbacher R, et al. Electrodiagnostic reference values for upper and lower limb nerve conduction studies in adult populations. Muscle Nerve 2016;54:371–7.

19. Andreu JL, Ly-Pen D, Millán I, et al. Local injection versus surgery in carpal tunnel syndrome: neurophysiologic outcomes of a randomized clinical trial. Clin Neurophysiol 2014;125:1479–84.

20. Armstrong T, Devor W, Borschel L, et al. Intracarpal steroid injection is safe and effective for short-term management of carpal tunnel syndrome. Muscle Nerve 2004;29(1):82–8.

21. American Academy of Orthopaedic Surgery (AAOS). Clinical practice guideline on the treatment of carpal tunnel syndrome. 2016.

22. Thompson JG. Diagnosis and treatment of carpal tunnel syndrome. Lancet Neurol 2017;16(4):263.

23. Padua L, Coraci D, Erra C, et al. Diagnosis and treatment of carpal tunnel syndrome – Authors' responses. Lancet Neurol 2017;16(4):263–4.

24. Lane LB, Starecki M, Olson A, et al. Carpal tunnel syndrome diagnosis and treatment: a survey of members of the American Society for Surgery of the Hand. J Hand Surg Am 2014;39(11):2161–87.

25. Yugueros P, Berger RA. Anatomy of the carpal tunnel. [Chapter 2]. In: Luchetti R, Amadio PC, editors. Carpal tunnel syndrome. Berlin: Springer; 2007. p. 10–2.

26. Ghasemi-Rad M, Nosair E, Vegh A, et al. A handy review of carpal tunnel syndrome: from anatomy to diagnosis and treatment. World J Radiol 2014;6(6): 284–300.

27. Dumitru D, Amato AA, Zwarts MJ. Electrodiagnostic medicine. 2nd edition. Philadelphia: Hanley & Belfus, Inc; 2002. p. 1047–61.

28. Gutmann L. Median-ulnar nerve communications and carpal tunnel syndrome. J Neurol Neurosurg Psychiatr 1977;40:982–6.

29. Ahadi T, Raissi GR, Yavari M, et al. Prevalence of ulnar-to-median nerve motor fiber anastomosis (Riché-Cannieu communicating branch) in hand: an electrophysiological study. Med J Islam Repub Iran 2016;30:324.

30. Seidel ME, Seidel GK, Hakopian D, et al. Electrodiagnostic evidence of Berrettini anastomosis. J Clin Neurophysiol 2018;35(2):133–7.

31. Szabo RM, Chidgey LK. Stress carpal tunnel pressure in patients with carpal tunnel syndrome. J Hand Surg 1989;14A(4):624–7.

32. Rydevik B, Lundborg G, Bragge U. Effects of graded compression on intraneural blood flow: an in vivo study on rabbit tibial nerve. J Hand Surg 1981;6(1):3–12.
33. Becker J, Nora DB, Gomes I, et al. An evaluation of gender, obesity, age and diabetes mellitus as risk factors for carpal tunnel syndrome. Clin Neurophysiol 2002; 113(9):1429–34.
34. Geoghegan JM, Clark DI, Bainbridge LC, et al. Risk factors in carpal tunnel syndrome. J Hand Surg Br 2004;29(4):315–20.
35. da Costa BR, Vieira ER. Risk factors for work-related musculoskeletal disorders: a systematic review of recent longitudinal studies. Am J Ind Med 2010;53(3): 285–323.
36. Katz JN, Larson MG, Sabra A, et al. Carpal tunnel syndrome diagnostic utility of history and physical examination findings. Ann Intern Med 1990;112:321–7.
37. Claes F, Kasius KM, Meulstee J, et al. The treatment in carpal tunnel syndrome: does distribution of sensory symptoms matter? J Neurol Sci 2014;344(1–2): 143–8.
38. Alfonso MI, Dzwierzynski W. Hoffman-Tinel sign, the reality. Phys Med Rehabil Clin N Am 1998;9:721–36.
39. Durkan JA. A new diagnostic test for carpal tunnel syndrome. J Bone Joint Surg Am 1991;3:535–8.
40. Cheng CJ, Mackinnon-Patterson B, Beck JL, et al. Scratch collapse test for evaluation of carpal and cubital tunnel syndrome. J Hand Surg Am 2008;33:1518–24.
41. Boland RA, Kiernan MC. Assessing the accuracy of a combination of clinical tests for identifying carpal tunnel syndrome. J Clin Neurosci 2009;16:929–33.
42. Nakamichi K, Tachibana S. The use of ultrasonography in detection of synovitis in carpal tunnel syndrome. J Hand Surg Br 1993;18(2):176–9.
43. Presazzi A, Bortolotto C, Madonia L, et al. Carpal tunnel: normal anatomy, anatomical variants and ultrasound technique. J Ultrasound 2011;14(1):40–6.
44. Merhar GL, Clark RA, Schneider HJ, et al. High-resolution computed tomography of the wrist in patients with carpal tunnel syndrome. Skeletal Radiol 1986;15(7): 549–52.
45. Malladi N, Micklesen PJ, Hou J, et al. Carpal tunnel syndrome: a retrospective review of the correlation between the combined sensory index and clinical outcome after carpal tunnel decompression. Muscle Nerve 2010;41(4):453–7.
46. Shi Q, MacDermid JC. Is surgical intervention more effective than non-surgical treatment for carpal tunnel syndrome? A systematic review. J Orthop Surg Res 2011;6:17.
47. Ono S, Clapham PJ, Chung KC. Optimal management of carpal tunnel syndrome. Int J Gen Med 2010;3:255–61.
48. Page MJ, Massy-Westropp N, O'Connor D, et al. Splinting for carpal tunnel syndrome. Cochrane Database Syst Rev 2012;(7):CD010003.
49. Bland JDP. Hydrodissection for treatment of carpal tunnel syndrome. Muscle Nerve 2018;57:4–5.
50. Ferry S, Pritchard T, Keenan J, et al. Estimating the prevalence of delayed median nerve conduction in the general population. Br J Rheumatol 1998;37(6):630–5.
51. Kronlage SC, Memendez ME. The benefit of carpal tunnel release in patients with electrodiagnostically moderate and severe disease. J Hand Surg Am 2015;40(3): 438–44.
52. Melvin JL, Johnson EW, Duran R. Electrodiagnosis after surgery for carpal tunnel syndrome. Arch Phys Med Rehabil 1968;49:502–7.
53. Bland JD. Do nerve conduction studies predict the outcome of carpal tunnel decompression? Muscle Nerve 2001;24(7):935–40.

54. Fowler JR, Munsch M, Huang WC, et al. Pre-operative electrodiagnostic testing predicts time to resolution of symptoms after carpal tunnel release. J Hand Surg Eur Vol 2016;41E(2):137–42.

55. Visser LH, Ngo Q, Sascha JM, et al. Effect of corticosteroid injection for carpal tunnel syndrome: a relation with electrodiagnostic severity. Clin Neurophysiol 2012;123:838–42.

56. Witt JC, Hentz JG, Stevens JC. Carpal tunnel syndrome with normal conduction studies. Muscle Nerve 2004;29(4):515–24.

57. Kimura J. The carpal tunnel syndrome; localization of conduction abnormalities within the distal segment of the median nerve. Brain 1979;102:619–35.

58. Azadeh A, Vasaghi A, Jalli R, et al. Comparison of inching method and ultrasonographic findings in the determination of median nerve entrapment site in carpal tunnel syndrome. Am J Phys Med Rehabil 2017;96(12):869–73.

59. Triki L, Zouari HG, Kammoun R, et al. A reappraisal of small-and large-fiber damage in carpal tunnel syndrome: new insights into the value of the EMLA test for improving diagnostic sensitivity. Neurophysiol Clin 2017;47:427–36.

60. Pope D, Tang P. Carpal tunnel syndrome and distal radius fractures. Hand Clin 2018;34:27–32.

61. US Department of Labor Bureau of Labor Statistics. Available at: http://www.bls.gov/news.release/osh2.t11.htm. Accessed January 3, 2018.

62. NIH Carpal Tunnel Syndrome Fact Sheet National Institute of Neurological Diseases and Stroke (NINDS). Available at: http://www.ninds.nih.gov/disorders/carpal_tunnel/detail_carpal_tunnel.htm. Accessed January 5, 2018.

Steering Peripheral Neuropathy Workup

Michele L. Arnold, MD, FAAPMR, FAANEM

KEYWORDS

- Peripheral neuropathy • Polyneuropathy • Etiologic workup • Pattern recognition

KEY POINTS

- Having diagnosed peripheral polyneuropathy, the astute neuromuscular physician proceeds with an informed and targeted etiologic investigation, which is paramount to guiding available treatment, rather than resigning immediately to palliative care strategies.
- Pattern recognition is a useful tool for investigating the underlying etiology of peripheral neuropathy, using Barohn and Amato's 3-6-10 approach to categorize into 10 distinct phenotypic patterns that inform a more targeted etiologic workup.
- Cryptogenic idiopathic neuropathy accounts for 25% of patients with peripheral neuropathy, yet after additional workup, a proportion can be attributed to hereditary forms, immunologic causes (acquired demyelinating polyneuropathies, eg, chronic inflammatory demyelination polyradiculoneuropathy and variants), paraproteinemia, or undiagnosed medical conditions.
- Diagnostic workup should be guided by history, examination, electrodiagnostic findings, laboratory testing, and additional assessment tools. A balanced view of cost, risk, and benefit enables clinicians to capitalize on the diagnostic clues to achieve not just a diagnosis, but clinical value.

INTRODUCTION

Physicians commonly encounter peripheral neuropathy regardless of specialty or subspecialty, owing to its prevalence in the general population of 1% to 3%, increasing to 7% in those older than 50.[1] Unfortunately, many of the known etiologies of polyneuropathy cause irreversible peripheral nerve pathology. Lured by the perception that little can be offered, time-pressured clinicians may fail to see value in the workup of peripheral neuropathy. Additionally, peripheral neuropathy may be erroneously diagnosed based solely on reported symptoms in the face of known risk factors and assumptions about causation. Among those referred to specialists, the etiology for 25% of patients with peripheral neuropathy remains elusive despite a careful search,

Disclosure: None.
Physical Medicine and Rehabilitation, Swedish Health Services, 1600 E. Jefferson, Suite 300, Seattle, WA 98122, USA
E-mail address: michele.arnold@swedish.org

Phys Med Rehabil Clin N Am 29 (2018) 761–776
https://doi.org/10.1016/j.pmr.2018.06.010

aptly ascribing the term "cryptogenic" to idiopathic neuropathy.[2] After additional workup, however, a proportion can be attributed to hereditary forms, immunologic causes (acquired demyelinating, eg, chronic inflammatory demyelination polyradiculoneuropathy [CIDP] and variants), paraproteinemia, or undiagnosed medical conditions.[2–4]

Learning to recognize the various clinical and electrodiagnostic patterns of peripheral neuropathy enables a targeted approach to etiologic investigation, and subsequently guides patient discussions of self-management, disease course, and prognosis. Moreover, as advancements in neuropathology and pharmacotherapy inform the many etiologies of polyneuropathy, it is imperative for clinicians to identify the underlying etiology to appropriately guide treatment options and prevent complications.

PATHOPHYSIOLOGY OF PERIPHERAL NEUROPATHY

Polyneuropathy refers to pathology affecting multiple peripheral nerves and involves the cell body, axon, myelin sheath, or a combination thereof. Regardless of the etiology of peripheral neuropathy, pathophysiology devolves into predictable patterns of response to injury: demyelination, axonal degeneration, or a combination of both.

Demyelination can have a focal segmental distribution, such as neurapraxia, when compression is insufficient to damage axons, yet leads to injury involving a focal segment of myelin, resulting in action potential failure (conduction block) or conduction velocity slowing. Typical examples include acute compression and chronic entrapment. Generalized demyelination results in conduction block and/or temporal dispersion in multiple nerves often asymmetrically and in anatomic locations outside common areas of compression/entrapment.

Axonal (Wallerian) degeneration, represented by axonotmesis and neurotmesis, results from prolonged, focal crush injury or transection resulting in disintegration and removal of axon and myelin distal to injury followed by an alteration of neural properties proximal to injury (so-called "dying back"), and ultimately, cell body death. Axonopathy also can be the result of toxic degeneration or a generalized insult to the peripheral nervous system.

Many conditions affect both peripheral nerve myelin and axon, but ultimately, Wallerian axonal degeneration represents the final common pathway of neuronal injury. With significant axonal loss, secondary demyelination occurs, and in cases of severe demyelination, axonal injury also occurs. Furthermore, acute conduction block, axonal loss of varying durations, and chronic muscle atrophy can all manifest as amplitude loss on motor conduction studies. In chronic polyneuropathy, this often obscures the initial distinguishing pathophysiologic features that might steer toward a specific underlying etiology, contributing to the diagnostic quandary.

ASSESSMENT OF PERIPHERAL NEUROPATHY
History

Because the diagnosis of peripheral neuropathy relies heavily on pattern recognition, a thorough history will provide initial clues[5]:

- Symptoms: onset, timing, character, severity, location/distribution and symmetry, course, exacerbating and relieving factors. Nocturnal foot and leg pain is a common complaint, yet not well understood. Many patients describe hypersensitive dysesthesias on contact with footwear or bed sheets.

Numbness can manifest as a dull or foreign sensation involving the ball of the forefoot, as if a sock is bunched/wrinkled. Burning pain may suggest small fiber involvement.

- Preceding illnesses, immunizations, trauma, or exposures can provide clues to inflammatory demyelinating, compression, or toxic neuropathies, respectively. Antecedent illness, vaccination, or surgery is implicated in 60% to 70% of patients with acute inflammatory demyelination polyradiculoneuropathy.[6] A trigger can be identified in fewer than 30% of patients with CIDP, but respiratory and other infections, vaccinations, surgeries, blood transfusions, and even intraarticular steroid injections have been reported. In addition, pregnancy and infection have been reported to precede 20% to 30% of cases of CIDP exacerbation/relapse.[6]
- Associated symptoms: atrophy, fatigue, poor endurance, muscle cramps or stiffness, gait difficulties.
- Functional history: ambulatory distance, falls, transitions from floor to standing, and difficulty with climbing stairs, dressing, operating fasteners (buttons, zippers), reaching overhead, lifting, running, or performing vocational or avocational tasks.
- Medication history: query neurotoxic drugs.
- Past medical and surgical history, with attention to risk factors (see **Table 3**).
- Family history: neurologic diseases, gait abnormalities (use of gait aides, orthotics), skeletal deformities (pes cavus, hammer toes, amputations, scoliosis), pedigree if needed.
- Developmental history, when applicable.
- Social history:
  - Occupational and avocational history, query potential exposures to neurotoxins
  - Overseas travel/residence (infectious, nutritional, and other risks)
  - US military or prisoner of war experience (Agent Orange exposure, immunizations, physical/nutritional stressors, potential risk for amyotrophic lateral sclerosis [ALS][7])
  - Other potential environmental exposures: alcohol, illicit drug use, city versus well water, dietary idiosyncrasies, zinc-based denture adhesive use, others
- Review of symptoms: weight loss, swallowing dysfunction, dysautonomia, endocrinopathy, anemia, skin and joint changes, others.

Physical Examination

Physical examination findings focus not solely on the neuromuscular examination, but also should screen for etiologic clues, and assess overall function and gait safety. A basic neuromuscular examination[5] with clinical pearls is presented in **Tables 1** and **2**.

Electrodiagnostic Testing

Large-fiber polyneuropathies can be confirmed via nerve conduction studies and needle electromyography (EMG). Sufficient number and location of nerves should be examined to determine the pattern (axonal vs demyelinating, motor vs sensory) and distribution (symmetry, proximal vs distal) of involvement. Axonopathy manifests as diminished sensory nerve action potentials (SNAP) and compound muscle action potential (CMAP) amplitudes without significant prolongation of distal latencies or slowing of conduction velocity unless axonal loss is severe (eg, <20%–30% of the lower limit of normal). Criteria for demyelination are well-outlined in published guidelines[8]

Table 1
Neuromusculoskeletal examination basics

Examination	Key Finding(s)
Gait and balance assessment	• Heel walk, toe walk • Monitor for pathology: steppage, vaulting, foot drop, ataxia, or Trendelenburg patterns • Single leg stance • Romberg • Tandem gait
Spine examination	• Reduced range of motion, Spurling, dural tension signs, such as straight leg raise, quadrant loading may provide clues regarding potential radiculopathy • Paraspinal atrophy, head drop, camptocormia may suggest axial myopathy or motor neuron disease
Sensory examination	• Vibration, proprioception (early loss in large-fiber neuropathies) • Pinprick (often stocking or stocking-glove distribution loss) • Temperature • Light touch • Monofilament testing (loss of protective sensation) • Two-point discrimination (may be useful in assessment of mononeuropathy)
Reflexes	• Muscle stretch/deep tendon reflexes • Pathologic reflexes (Babinski, Hoffman, jaw jerk, others)

Examination	Key Finding(s)	Suggestions Re: Underlying Etiology
Extremities	• Contractures • Tinel, Phalen, or other provocative maneuvers • Palpation for enlarged peripheral nerves (superficial fibular, superficial radial, posterior auricular, others) • Foot drop (heel walk) • Ankle plantarflexion weakness (strength examination should include heel raises in single leg stance). Measuring limb circumference can provide objective assessment of calf (or thigh) atrophy.	• Nonspecific • Compression or entrapment neuropathy • Hereditary neuropathies • Amyloidosis • Acquired demyelinating polyneuropathies • L5 (L4) radiculopathy • Fibular neuropathy • Sciatic neuropathy involving fibular division • Charcot-Marie-Tooth • Motor neuron disease • Distal myopathies • S1 radiculopathy • Sciatic neuropathy • Proximal tibial neuropathy • Severe peripheral neuropathies • Motor neuron disease

(continued on next page)

Table 1
(continued)

Examination	Key Finding(s)	Suggestions Re: Underlying Etiology
Foot examination	• Metatarsalgia (due to distal migration of metatarsal fat pad resulting from intrinsic atrophy and shortening of interossei and lumbricals, resulting in acquired hammertoe deformities)	• Nonspecific
	• Hypertrophic callouses or ulcerations	• Nonspecific • Diabetes • Peripheral vascular disease
	• Intrinsic atrophy, pes cavus, hammertoe deformities, Charcot arthropathy • Atrophy of forelegs ("inverted champagne bottle" shape)	• Hereditary sensory motor neuropathy (HSMN) • Charcot-Marie-Tooth
Shoulder girdle examination	• Atrophy • Static and/or dynamic scapular winging	• Cervical radiculopathy • Brachial plexopathy and Parsonage-Turner syndrome • Proximal mononeuropathies (long thoracic, dorsal scapular, or spinal accessory neuropathies) • Motor neuron disease
Hip examination	• Hip or thigh weakness • Knee buckling	• Lumbosacral radiculopathy • Lumbosacral plexopathy • Radiculoplexus neuropathy • Femoral/proximal mononeuropathy
Cranial nerves	• Facial symmetry • Pupillary responses • Eyelid strength • Vocal quality and volume • Inspection of tongue for atrophy or fasciculations	• Bell palsy • Facial neuropathy • Junctional disorders • Motor neuron disease
	• Axial strength (eg, neck flexors and extensors)	• Axial myopathy • Motor neuron disease

Data from McDonald CM. Clinical approach to the diagnostic evaluation of hereditary and acquired neuromuscular diseases. Phys Med Rehabil Clin N Am 2012;23(3):495–563.

but generally manifest as prolonged distal sensory and motor latencies and slow conduction velocities, with conduction block and temporal dispersion. Proximal conduction studies such as F-waves, H-reflexes, and blink reflexes can be helpful adjuncts.

Table 2
Other physical examination pearls

System	Finding	Suggestions Re: Underlying Etiology
Respiratory	• Dyspnea on exertion	• Motor neuron disease • Acute inflammatory demyelinating polyradiculoneuropathy (AIDP)
	• Asymmetric diaphragmatic excursion (hemidiaphragm paralysis)	• Phrenic neuropathy • Parsonage-Turner syndrome involving phrenic nerve • AIDP
Cardiovascular	• Heart rate variability • Peripheral pulses • Capillary refill	• Autonomic neuropathy • Peripheral arterial disease
Skin	• Extremities: cool temperature, pallor, hair loss, onychomycosis • Rash, telangiectasia • Clubbing • Mees lines	• Peripheral arterial disease • Vasculitis, collagen vascular disease • Cardiopulmonary disease • Arsenic neuropathy
Lymphatic	• Lymphadenopathy	• Neoplastic disease • Paraproteinemia • Amyloidosis

Data from McDonald CM. Clinical approach to the diagnostic evaluation of hereditary and acquired neuromuscular diseases. Phys Med Rehabil Clin N Am 2012;23(3):495–563.

When examination findings are mild or moderate, nerve conduction studies should focus on the more involved limb, whereas they should focus on the least involved limb when examination findings suggest more severe disease.

Donofrio and Albers[8] recommend a peripheral neuropathy protocol consisting of fibular (extensor digitorum brevis), tibial (abductor hallucis), ulnar (hypothenar), and median (thenar) CMAPs with corresponding F-waves, sural (averaged if needed) and median SNAPs, followed by corresponding nerves on the contralateral limb if abnormal. Facial or blink reflex studies may be considered if cranial nerve involvement is suspected. Needle EMG should include tibialis anterior, medial gastrocnemius, lumbar paraspinal muscles, possibly foot intrinsic muscles, and first dorsal interosseous (hand), followed by at least one contralateral muscle if any of the aforementioned are abnormal. Needle EMG is a pivotal component to evaluate for motor axonal loss, degree of denervation, and pattern of involvement and helps rule out competing diagnoses, such as radiculopathy(ies), myopathy, and other mimics of polyneuropathy (eg, motor neuron disease, others).

The electrodiagnostic evaluation of motor neuron disease merits additional mention largely outside of the scope of this discussion; however, the reader should reference both the revised El Escorial[9] and Awaji[10] electrodiagnostic criteria for ALS, as well as a more recent publication outlining optimal muscle selection for needle EMG in ALS.[11]

Similarly, strict compliance with published evidence-based diagnostic criteria is paramount to confirm the diagnosis of CIDP, because one-third of patients with CIDP in the United States have reportedly been incorrectly diagnosed and possibly receiving inappropriate treatment.[12] Refer to **Box 1** for the European Federation of Neurologic Societies and Peripheral Nerve Society electrodiagnostic criteria for the diagnosis of CIDP.[13]

Box 1

EFNS/PNS electrodiagnostic criteria for chronic inflammatory demyelination polyradiculoneuropathy

Definite: at least 1 of the following:
- Prolongation of the DML ≥50% above the ULN in 2 nerves.
- Reduction in motor NCV ≥30% below the LLN in 2 nerves.
- Prolongation of F-wave minimal latency ≥30% above the ULN in 2 nerves (≥50% above the ULN if the distal CMAP amplitude is <80% of the LLN).
- Absence of F-waves in 2 nerves if their distal CMAP amplitudes are ≥20% of the LLN and at least 1 other demyelinating parameter in at least 1 other nerve.
- Partial motor conduction block in 2 nerves:
  - ≥50% amplitude reduction of the proximal relative to the distal CMAP, if the distal CMAP is ≥20% of the LLN
  - OR in 1 nerve AND at least 1 other demyelinating parameter in at least 1 other nerve.
- Abnormal temporal dispersion in ≥2 nerves (>30% duration increase between the proximal and distal CMAP).
- Prolonged distal CMAP duration in at least 1 nerve AND at least 1 other demyelinating parameter in at least 1 other nerve.

Probable: ≥30% amplitude reduction of the proximal relative to the distal CMAP in 2 nerves if the distal CMAP amplitude is ≥20% of the LLN, OR in 1 nerve AND at least 1 other demyelinating parameter in at least 1 other nerve.

Possible: as in the definite category, but in only 1 nerve.

Several investigators have expressed concern with this classification because of low specificity.

Abbreviations: CMAP, compound muscle action potential; DML, distal motor latency; EFNS, European Federation of Neurologic Societies; LLN, lower limit of normal; NCV, nerve conduction velocity; PNS, Peripheral Nerve Society; ULN, upper limit of normal.
Data from Joint Task Force of the EFNS and the PNS. European Federation of Neurological Societies/Peripheral Nerve Society Guideline on management of chronic inflammatory demyelinating polyradiculoneuropathy: report of a joint task force of the European Federation of Neurological Societies and the Peripheral Nerve Society–First Revision. J Peripher Nerv Syst 2010;15:1–9.

ETIOLOGY

Having diagnosed peripheral polyneuropathy, the astute neuromuscular physician proceeds with an informed and targeted etiologic investigation. The identification of etiology(ies) is paramount to guiding available treatment, rather than resigning immediately to palliative care strategies.

Neuromuscular medicine consultants fall into 2 polar groups: (1) "pragmatists" who aim to solve the clinical problem with minimal investigation, and (2) "completists" who seek to eliminate every possibility, however remote it may be, even when lacking therapeutic relevance. Pragmatists may miss rarities, whereas completists risk overuse of resources and even misdiagnosis if misled by false-positive results. It is important to maintain a balanced view and capitalize on the diagnostic clues to achieve not just a diagnosis, but clinical value. In other words, *"do the right thing and not everything."*[14]

The diagnostic workup should be guided by history, examination, and electrodiagnostic findings, given the wide spectrum of etiologic considerations. Much has been published in recent years regarding pattern recognition as a tool for sleuthing out the etiology of peripheral neuropathy.[3,15–17]

Barohn and Amato[3] suggest a *3-6-10 approach*, characterized by 3 goals and 6 key questions, leading to 10 phenotypic patterns facilitating a narrowed and refined diagnostic workup.

3 Goals[3]:
1. Determine anatomic and physiologic locations.
2. Determine etiology.
3. Determine treatment.

6 Key Questions help guide and inform the previous goals 1 and 2[3]:
1. What *systems* are involved?
   - Motor
   - Sensory
   - Autonomic
   - Mixed
2. What is the *distribution* of weakness?
   - Distal-only versus proximal and distal?
   - Focal, asymmetric, or symmetric?
3. What is the nature of the *sensory* involvement?
   - Severe pain/burning or stabbing
   - Proprioceptive loss
4. Is there evidence of *upper motor neuron* involvement?
   - With sensory loss?
   - Without sensory loss?
5. What is the *temporal* evolution?
   - Acute (days to 4 weeks)
   - Subacute (4–8 weeks)
   - Chronic (>8 weeks)
   - Preceding events, drugs, toxins?
6. Is there evidence for a *hereditary* neuropathy?
   - Family history
   - Skeletal deformities
   - Signs > symptoms

10 Distinct Phenotypic Patterns have been outlined:
   The distinct clinical features of each pattern enable the neuromuscular physician to not only recognize the various patterns of presentation, but customize further diagnostic testing to confirm the clinical impression. (Note: although it is less-frequently encountered than pattern 2, pattern 1 is listed sequentially first to highlight the importance of not missing the associated conditions because they are often amenable to immunotherapy.) There is level C evidence that screening laboratory studies be considered for patients with polyneuropathy.[18] Laboratory and additional diagnostic workup should be targeted based on clinical and electrodiagnostic findings.[18] A recommended laboratory assessment of each phenotypic pattern is listed in tandem in **Table 3**.

Additional Assessment Tools

Neuromuscular applications for *diagnostic ultrasound* are expanding beyond the assessment of entrapment neuropathy, now including assessment of optimal muscle for biopsy, fasciculations, atrophy, and conditions associated with peripheral nerve enlargement (CIDP, Charcot-Marie-Tooth [CMT], hereditary neuropathy with liability to pressure palsies [HNPP], amyloid).[20]

   Peripheral nerve biopsy can be useful in the setting of asymmetric neuropathy with sensory loss and weakness, and particularly in the evaluation of suspected

Table 3
Ten phenotypical patterns and recommended laboratory workup

Etiologies	Suggested Laboratory Workup
Pattern 1: Symmetric proximal and distal weakness with sensory loss	

Consider:
• Inflammatory demyelinating polyneuropathy (Guillain-Barré syndrome/acute inflammatory demyelinating polyradiculoneuropathy, chronic inflammatory demyelination polyradiculoneuropathy, and variants)
• Confirm diagnosis using published clinical criteria and electrodiagnostic criteria for demyelination[12]
	Consider specialty screenings:
	• Serologies:
	  ○ *Campylobacter jejuni*
	  ○ Hepatitis
	  ○ Influenza
	  ○ Cytomegalovirus
	  ○ *Mycoplasma pneumoniae*
	  ○ Epstein-Barr virus
	  ○ Human immunodeficiency virus (HIV)
	  ○ Rapid plasma reagin (RPR) for syphilis
	  ○ Others
	• Autoantibodies[19]:
	  ○ Anti-MAG, anti-sulfatide: neuropathies associated with paraproteinemia
	  ○ Anti-GM1: Multifocal motor neuropathy, AMAN
	  ○ Anti-GQ1b: Miller-Fisher syndrome
	  ○ Others

Pattern 2: Symmetric distal sensory loss with or without distal weakness	

Consider:
• Cryptogenic (idiopathic) sensory polyneuropathy
• Metabolic disorders[6]
  ○ Vitamin deficiencies (B12, folate, thiamine, vitamin E)
  ○ Malabsorption: bariatric and gastric surgeries, inflammatory bowel disease
  ○ Renal disease
  ○ Chronic liver disease
  ○ Metabolic syndrome
• Drugs[16]:
  ○ Neurologic/psychiatric agents: phenytoin, amitriptyline, lithium
  ○ Antimicrobials: nitrofurantoin, metronidazole, chloramphenicol, tuberculosis therapies, chloroquine, hydroxychloroquine
  ○ Cardiovascular agents: statins, amiodarone, flecainide, hydralazine
  ○ Nitrous oxide
  ○ Antirheumatic agents: colchicine, gold, leflunomide, methotrexate
  ○ Immunomodulators: tacrolimus, interferon-α, ipilimumab, nivolumab, pembrolizumab, bortezomib, others
  ○ Antineoplastic therapies: various chemotherapeutic agents, paclitaxel and other taxanes, vinca alkaloids, platinum analogues, doxorubicin, etoposide, ifosfamide, misonidazole
  ○ Antinucleosides
	Highest yield[18]:
	• Fasting blood sugar; if negative then glucose tolerance test
	• Serum B12 with metabolites (methylmalonic acid with/without homocysteine)
	• SPEP with immunofixation, UPEP, +/− quantitative immunoglobulins
	
	Additional laboratory tests to consider:
	• Erythrocyte sedimentation rate
	• C-reactive protein
	• Rheumatoid factor (RF)
	• Antinuclear antibody (ANA)
	• Thyroid stimulating hormone with reflexive T4
	• Complete blood count with differential
	• Complete metabolic panel
	• Serum folate
	• Heavy metals from serum and/or 24-h urine

(continued on next page)

Table 3
(continued)

Etiologies	Suggested Laboratory Workup

• Toxinsx[16]:
  ○ Alcoholism
  ○ Heavy metal toxicity: lead, arsenic, inorganic mercury, zinc, thallium, gold others
  ○ Herbicides (dichlorophenoxyacetic acid, Agent Orange, and other deforestation agents)
  ○ Organophosphate insecticides/pesticides (parathion, dioxin, others)
  ○ Industrial agents: acrylamide, polychlorinated biphenyl, vinyl chloride (used to make polyvinyl chloride plastic and vinyl products)
  ○ Solvents: n-hexane (glue sniffing) and other hexacarbons, dry-cleaning solvents, carbon disulfide, perchloroethylene, trichloroethylene, triorthocresyl phosphate, ethylene oxide, styrene, toluene, methyl n-butyl ketone, mixed solvents, and others
• Endocrinopathy[6]:
  ○ Diabetes mellitus
  ○ Thyroid disease
  ○ Acromegaly
• Hereditary*: Charcot-Marie-Tooth (CMT), amyloidosis and others
• Systemic disorders[6]:
  ○ Peripheral arterial disease
  ○ Monoclonal gammopathy/paraproteinemia
  ○ Amyloidosis
  ○ POEMS (polyneuropathy, organomegaly, endocrinopathy, monoclonal protein, skin abnormalities)
  ○ Sarcoidosis
  ○ Collagen vascular diseases
  ○ Critical illness
	*There is level A evidence for genetic testing in patients with suspected hereditary neuropathy and level C evidence in patents with cryptogenic polyneuropathy who exhibit a hereditary neuropathy phenotype[18]:
	• Charcot-Marie-Tooth 1A: assay for PMP22 duplication
	• Hereditary neuropathy with liability to pressure palsies (HNPP): assay for PMP22 deletion
	• X-linked Charcot-Marie-Tooth: Next-Generation sequencing for connexin-32
	• Charcot-Marie-Tooth 2A: Next-Generation sequencing for mitofusin 2

Pattern 3: Asymmetric distal weakness with sensory loss

Multiple nerves, consider:
• Vasculitis (various collagen vascular/connective tissue disorders)[6]:
  ○ Polyarteritis nodosa
  ○ Churg-Strauss syndrome
  ○ Wegener granulomatosis
  ○ Temporal arteritis
  ○ Rheumatoid arthritis
  ○ Systemic lupus erythematosus
  ○ Sjögren's syndrome
	• RF, anti-cyclic citrullinated peptide antibody
	• ANA panel (anti-double-stranded DNA (dsDNA), anti-Sm, SS-A (Ro), SS-B (La), anti-RNP, anti-Jo, anti-centromere, Scl-70, others as indicated)
	• Anticytoplasmic antibodies: p-ANCA, c-ANCA
	• Cryoglobulins
	• Serum complement
	• Lyme titer

(continued on next page)

Table 3 *(continued)*	
Etiologies	**Suggested Laboratory Workup**
○ Scleroderma ○ Cryoglobulinemia ○ Others • HNPP • Multifocal acquired demyelinating sensory and motor (MADSAM) neuropathy • Infectious (leprosy, Lyme, sarcoid, HIV) Single nerves/regions, consider: • Compressive mononeuropathy • Radiculopathy • Herpes zoster focal paresis	• HIV
Pattern 4: Asymmetric proximal and distal weakness with sensory loss	
Consider[3]: • Polyradiculopathy • Radiculoplexus neuropathy (neurogenic amyotrophy) • Meningeal carcinomatosis or lymphomatosis • Sarcoidosis • Amyloidosis • Lyme disease • Hereditary (HNPP, familial) • Idiopathic	• Imaging studies as appropriate • Lyme titer • HNPP: assay for PMP22 deletion • Biopsy, as appropriate
Pattern 5: Asymmetric distal weakness without sensory loss	
With upper motor neuron findings, consider[3]: • Motor neuron disease: ○ Amyotrophic lateral sclerosis (ALS) ○ Primary lateral sclerosis (PLS) Without upper motor neuron findings, consider: • Progressive muscular atrophy (PMA) • Multifocal motor neuropathy (MMN) • Multifocal acquired motor axonopathy (MAMA) • Juvenile monomelic amyotrophy	• Complete blood count, CMP • Thyroid function tests • C-reactive protein • Creatine kinase • Serum copper • Serum B12 with metabolites (methylmalonic acid) • SPEP, UPEP, immunofixation • ANA • RPR; FTA-ABS (treponemal assay antibody *Treponema pallidum*) • HIV • Consider: ○ Lyme titer ○ Anti-GM1 antibody ○ Genetic testing for familial ALS (C9orf72, SOD-1, others) or Kennedy disease ○ Hexosaminidase A
Pattern 6: Symmetric sensory loss and distal areflexia with UMN findings	
Consider[3]: • B12 deficiency • Copper deficiency (including zinc toxicity) • Other causes of combined system degeneration with peripheral neuropathy • Inherited disorders ○ Adrenomyeloneuropathy ○ Metachromatic leukodystrophy	• Serum B12 with metabolites (methylmalonic acid with/without homocysteine) • Serum vitamin E • Serum copper • Serum zinc • RPR; FTA-ABS

(continued on next page)

Table 3
(continued)

Etiologies	Suggested Laboratory Workup
○ Friedreich ataxia	

Pattern 7: Symmetric weakness without sensory loss*

* Some overlap with myopathy and NMJ disorders[3] • Proximal and distal weakness: consider spinal muscular atrophy • Distal weakness: consider hereditary motor neuropathy	• Creatine kinase • Aldolase • Muscle biopsy • Anti-acetylcholine receptor antibodies • Myositis-specific antibodies

Pattern 8: Focal midline proximal symmetric weakness*

* Some overlap with myopathy NMJ disorders. Consider[3]:
 • Neck extensor weakness
   ○ Isolated neck extensor myopathy
   ○ Axial myopathy
   ○ ALS
 • Bulbar weakness
   ○ ALS
   ○ PLS
	• Creatine kinase
	 • Aldolase
	 • Muscle biopsy
	 • Myositis-specific antibodies
	 • Consider other studies as listed under pattern 5

Pattern 9: Asymmetric proprioceptive sensory loss without weakness

Consider[3]:
 • Sensory neuronopathy (ganglionopathy):
   ○ Cancer
   ○ Paraneoplastic syndromes (small-cell lung cancer, lymphoma, multiple myeloma, others)
   ○ Sjögren's syndrome
   ○ Idiopathic sensory neuronopathy
   ○ Cisplatinum and other analogues
   ○ Vitamin B6 toxicity
   ○ HIV-related sensory neuronopathy
 • Chronic immune sensory polyradiculopathy (CISP)
	• Routine cancer screenings
	 • Paraneoplastic panel (anti-Hu, others)
	 • Serum B6
	 • HIV
	 • ANA reflexive panel: anti-dsDNA, anti-Sm, SS-A (Ro), SS-B (La), anti-RNP, anti-Jo, anti-centromere, Scl-70, others as indicated
	 • Anticytoplasmic antibodies: p-ANCA, c-ANCA

Pattern 10: Autonomic symptoms and signs

Consider: neuropathies associated with autonomic dysfunction[3]: • Hereditary sensory autonomic neuropathy • Diabetes mellitus • Amyloidosis (familial and acquired) • Guillain-Barré syndrome • Vincristine-induced • Porphyria • HIV-related autonomic neuropathy • Idiopathic pandysautonomia	• Fasting blood sugar; if negative then glucose tolerance test • SPEP with immunofixation, UPEP, +/− quantitative immunoglobulins • HIV

Abbreviations: AMAN, acute motor axonal neuropathy; Anti-Sm, autoantibodies against smith antigen; CMP, comprehensive metabolic panel; GM, antibodies to ganglioside GM1; MAG, myelin-associated glycoprotein; NMJ, neuromuscular junction; SPEP, serum protein electrophoresis; UPEP, urine protein electrophoresis; UM, upper motor neuron.

Data from Barohn RJ, Amato AA. Pattern recognition approach to neuropathy and neuronopathy. Neurol Clin 2013;31(2):343–61; and England JD, Gronseth G, Franklin GT, et al. Practice parameter evaluation of distal symmetric polyneuropathy: role of laboratory and genetic testing (an evidence-based review). Muscle Nerve 2009;72:116–25.

amyloid neuropathy, mononeuropathy multiplex due to vasculitis, demyelinating polyneuropathy (including atypical forms of CIDP), hereditary neuropathy, and leprosy.[21,22] Literature is insufficient to recommend nerve biopsy for acquired, distal, symmetric, or length-dependent peripheral neuropathies.[22]

Epidermal nerve fiber density testing via skin punch biopsy is a validated technique with level C evidence in the workup of small fiber neuropathy and potentially amyloidosis.[22]

There is level B evidence in support of the use of validated *autonomic testing* (R-R interval variation, sympathetic skin response, thermoregulatory sweat test, quantitative sudomotor axon reflex test, or others) for suspected autonomic neuropathies.[22]

Disease Progression

Disease trajectory is variable and hinges on the course of the underlying etiology. A minority of the listed etiologies are potentially treatable (most notably immune-mediated demyelinating neuropathies), and fewer still are reversible. Acute neuropathies, such as Guillain-Barré syndrome, may appear suddenly, progress rapidly, and resolve subacutely. Treatment of underlying etiologies is paramount and often requires collaboration among treating practitioners. Underlying endocrine conditions should be addressed and medical treatments titrated to achieve optimal control. In diabetic individuals, glycemic control is pivotal, with goal HbA1c <6.5% to 7.0%, fasting/preprandial capillary plasma glucose 80 to 130 mg/dL, and peak postprandial glucose less than 180.[23] Thyroid replacement therapy should be optimized, although ideal target thyroid hormone levels remain disputed.

Most chronic forms of peripheral polyneuropathy are subtly progressive over many years. Slow, predictable decline in a patient with known neuropathy can be accelerated by the development of new medical conditions that have neurologic manifestations (eg, multifactorial neuropathy), or exacerbated by various infections, surgeries, or illnesses.

In subacute and chronic cases, palliative care becomes the primary goal of treatment, focusing on symptomatic control. Even the most efficacious medications provide moderate relief in 50% to 60% of patients, and there is only a 20% probability of complete pain relief with a single prescription. This leads practitioners to pursue combination therapy; however, there are no proven polypharmacy algorithms.[24]

Associated Conditions and Complications

Loss of sensation, and particularly proprioception, causes sensory ataxic gait and increased risk of a fall, more so when accompanied by leg weakness or foot drop. Loss of protective sensation can result in neuropathic ulceration or Charcot joint deformities. Autonomic neuropathies can cause impaired thermoregulation, gastrointestinal dysmotility, neurogenic bladder, sexual dysfunction, heart rate and blood pressure dysregulation, and exercise intolerance. Peripheral neuropathies associated with peripheral nerve enlargement (CIDP, CMT, HNPP) or deposition (amyloid) may present with entrapment mononeuropathies or even manifest as polyradiculopathy or neurogenic claudication.

Prognosis

Determining the underlying etiology can guide discussions of treatment as well as prognosis. Peripheral neuropathy outcomes are as varied as their etiologies. Critical illness neuropathy, for example, portends chronic disability and increased hospital mortality, whereas acquired demyelinating neuropathies respond favorably to immunotherapy. In general, neuropathies with extensive axonal loss, denervation, and atrophy have a poor prognosis for full recovery. Loss of monofilament sensation can predict neuropathic ulceration in diabetic neuropathy.[25] Because many forms of neuropathy are slowly progressive or stable, palliative therapies often become the mainstay of treatment.

In chronic cases, appropriate steps should be taken to prevent complications. Loss of protective sensation prompts the need for routine foot care and skin checks. Proprioceptive loss and imbalance can be ameliorated with gait aides and fall-prevention strategies. When ankle dorsiflexion weakness is identified, ankle foot orthoses can significantly improve gait function and prevent falls and ankle injuries. Static orthoses may play a role in contracture prevention. Therapeutic exercise can maintain and improve strength, endurance, coordination, balance, agility, flexibility, and range of motion, and may reduce perceived pain interference, but imparts no direct benefit on neurologic recovery.[26,27]

Patient and Family Education

Patients with hereditary neuropathy should specifically be counseled regarding risk to future family members and avoiding common exacerbating factors and neurotoxic medications.

Providers should educate patients and families regarding skin and foot care, burn prevention, impact from possible autonomic dysfunction, as well as the prognosis and course of their condition. Patients should be reassured that physical activity will not cause neurologic decline or progression of disease, but may exacerbate neuropathic symptoms. Fall-prevention skills should be outlined, including a higher fall risk in low-light conditions (due to lack of visual inputs for balance) and on uneven and unfamiliar surfaces.

Underlying cause(s) of peripheral neuropathy and potential exacerbating factors should be identified and mitigated. Providers should adhere to recommended treatment guidelines, and clearly communicate treatment goals. Treatment risks should be minimized with appropriate titration and dose adjustment, reassessment of ongoing need, routine follow-up, and laboratory monitoring when indicated.

Fall risk should be assessed in all patients with peripheral neuropathy, and appropriate preventive measures implemented.

SUMMARY

Patients rely on clinicians to (1) conduct a cost-effective etiologic workup, (2) render an informed diagnosis, and (3) provide education regarding disease progression, prognosis, treatment, and management/prevention of complications. Beyond knowledge and skill, this demands curiosity and tenacity on the part of the neuromuscular clinician. Use of pattern recognition using Barohn and Amato's 3-6-10 approach narrows the differential to 1 of 10 distinct phenotypic patterns, informing a targeted etiologic workup. Equipped with the underlying etiology of peripheral neuropathy, clinicians can customize treatment and patient education. Few of the known etiologies of peripheral neuropathy are fully reversible, and therefore, management should include ongoing surveillance for conditions that can secondarily exacerbate the known underlying condition. Shared patient-physician decision making should drive selection of palliative pharmacotherapy for dysesthesias. Even among the 25% with cryptogenic peripheral neuropathy, clinicians can provide patient value beyond simply palliating neuropathic pain. Partnering with patients to provide education, set expectations, and lay out a plan for self-management provides opportunity to improve patient-reported outcomes and patient satisfaction, and reduce consumption of redundant resources in search of an elusive cure. Addressing impairments in daily functioning, sleep, and health-related quality of life have the potential to ameliorate the humanistic and economic burden of peripheral neuropathy.[28]

REFERENCES

1. Hanewinckel R, van Oijen M, Ikram MA, et al. The epidemiology and risk factors of chronic polyneuropathy. Eur J Epidemiol 2016;31:5–20.
2. Dyck PJ, Oviatt KF, Lambert EH. Intensive evaluation of referred unclassified neuropathies yields improved diagnosis. Ann Neurol 1981;10(3):222–6.
3. Barohn RJ, Amato AA. Pattern recognition approach to neuropathy and neuronopathy. Neurol Clin 2013;31(2):343–61.
4. Singer MA, Vernino SA, Wolfe GI. Idiopathic neuropathy: new paradigms, new promise. J Peripher Nerv Syst 2012;17(Suppl 2):43–9.
5. McDonald CM. Clinical approach to the diagnostic evaluation of hereditary and acquired neuromuscular diseases. Phys Med Rehabil Clin N Am 2012;23(3): 495–563.
6. Amato AA, Dumitru D. Acquired neuropathies. In: Dumitru D, Amato AA, Zwarts M, editors. Electrodiagnostic medicine. 2nd edition. Philadelphia: Hanley & Belfus; 2001. p. 937–60.
7. Beard JD, Kamel F. Military service, deployments, and exposures in relation to amyotrophic lateral sclerosis etiology and survival. Epidemiol Rev 2015;37: 55–70.
8. Donofrio PD, Albers JW. AAEM minimonograph 34: polyneuropathy: classification by nerve conduction studies and electromyography. Muscle Nerve 1990;13: 889–903.
9. Brooks BR, Miller RG, Swash M, et al, for the World Federation of Neurology Research Committee on Motor Neuron Diseases. El Escorial revisited: revised criteria for the diagnosis of amyotrophic lateral sclerosis. Amyotroph Lateral Scler 2000;1:293–300.
10. Geevasinga N, Loy CT, Menon P, et al. Awaji criteria improves the diagnostic sensitivity in amyotrophic lateral sclerosis: a systematic review using individual patient data. Clin Neurophysiol 2016;127:2684–91.
11. Babu S, Pioro EP, Li J, et al. Optimizing muscle selection for electromyography in amyotrophic lateral sclerosis. Muscle Nerve 2017;56(1):36–44.
12. Cornblath DR, Gorson KC, Hughes RA, et al. Observations on chronic inflammatory demyelinating polyneuropathy: a plea for a rigorous approach to diagnosis and treatment. J Neurol Sci 2013;330:2–3.
13. Joint Task Force of the EFNS and the PNS. European Federation of Neurological Societies/Peripheral Nerve Society Guideline on management of chronic inflammatory demyelinating polyradiculoneuropathy: report of a joint task force of the European Federation of Neurological Societies and the Peripheral Nerve Society–First Revision. J Peripher Nerv Syst 2010;15:1–9.
14. Misra UK, Kalita J, Nair PP. Diagnostic approach to peripheral neuropathy. Ann Indian Acad Neurol 2008;11(2):89–97.
15. Dyck PJ, Dyck JB, Grant IA, et al. Ten steps in characterizing and diagnosing patients with peripheral neuropathy. Neurology 1996;47:10–7.
16. Pestronk A. Polyneuropathy differential diagnosis. Washington University St. Louis Neuromuscular Disease Center; 2015. Available at: http://neuromuscular. wustl.edu/naltbrain.html. Accessed January 14, 2017.

17. Poncelet AN. An algorithm for the evaluation of peripheral neuropathy. Am Fam Physician 1998;57(4):755–64.

18. England JD, Gronseth G, Franklin GT, et al. Practice parameter evaluation of distal symmetric polyneuropathy: role of laboratory and genetic testing (an evidence-based review). Muscle Nerve 2009;72:116–25.

19. Emilien D, Hugh W. Diagnostic utility of auto antibodies in inflammatory nerve disorders. J Neuromuscul Dis 2015;2(2):107–12.

20. Hobson-Webb LD. Neuromuscular ultrasound in polyneuropathies and motor neuron disease. Muscle Nerve 2013;47:790–804.

21. Said G. Indications and usefulness of nerve biopsy. Arch Neurol 2002;59(10): 1532–9.

22. England JD, Gronseth G, Franklin GT, et al. Practice parameter: the evaluation of distal symmetric polyneuropathy: the role of autonomic testing, nerve biopsy, and skin biopsy (an evidence-based review). Report of the American Academy of Neurology, the American Association of Neuromuscular and Electrodiagnostic Medicine, and the American Academy of Physical Medicine and Rehabilitation. PM R 2009;1(1):14–22.

23. American Diabetes Association Standards of Medical Care in Diabetes. Glycemic targets. Diabetes Care 2017;40(Suppl 1):S48–56.

24. Cohen K, Shinkazh N, Frank J, et al. Pharmacological treatment of diabetic peripheral neuropathy. P T 2015;40(6):372–88.

25. Paisey RB, Darby T, George AM, et al. Prediction of protective sensory loss, neuropathy and foot ulceration in type 2 diabetes. BMJ Open Diabetes Res Care 2016;4:e000163.

26. Dombovy ML. Rehabilitation management of neuropathies. In: Dyck PJ, Thomas PK, editors. Peripheral neuropathy. 4th edition. Philadelphia: Elsevier; 2005. p. 2621–36.

27. Yoo M, D'Silva LJ, Martin K. Pilot study of exercise therapy on painful diabetic peripheral neuropathy. Pain Med 2015;16:1482–9.

28. Alleman CJ, Westerhout KY, Hensen M, et al. Humanistic and economic burden of painful diabetic peripheral neuropathy in Europe: a review of the literature. Diabetes Res Clin Pract 2015;109(2):215–25.

Elucidating the Cause of Pelvic Pain

Andrew Dubin, MD, MS

KEYWORDS

- Chronic pelvic pain • Flexion, abduction, external rotation
- Posterior pelvic pain provocation test

KEY POINTS

- Chronic pelvic pain is a common condition.
- Establishing a diagnosis can be complicated by the interplay between various organ systems, including urologic, gynecologic, gastrointestinal, neurologic, endocrinological, psychological, and musculoskeletal.
- Frequently, the patient will have seen multiple providers and undergone multiple tests, as well as invasive procedures, before the musculoskeletal system is even considered in the differential diagnosis.
- Typically, the musculoskeletal and nervous systems become suspected culprits only once all other potential etiologies have been eliminated.

INTRODUCTION TO THE PROBLEM

Chronic pelvic pain is a common condition, and often represents the final focal point for many patients who present to urologists, obstetric/gynecological physicians, colorectal surgeons, gastroenterologists, urogynecologists, orthopedic surgeons, and physiatrists, to name but a few physician specialties. In many instances, the etiology is never clearly elucidated.[1] Establishing a diagnosis can be complicated by the interplay between various organ systems, including urologic, gynecologic, gastrointestinal, neurologic, endocrinological, psychological, and musculoskeletal. Frequently the patient will have seen multiple providers and undergone multiple tests and invasive procedures before the musculoskeletal system is even considered in the differential diagnosis. Typically, the musculoskeletal and nervous systems become suspected culprits only once all other potential etiologies have been eliminated.

PRESENTATION

A major complicating factor that needs to be overcome is patient reluctance to discuss issues of chronic pelvic pain with physicians. Additionally, many physicians

Disclosure: The author has nothing to disclose.
Department of Physical Medicine and Rehabilitation, Albany Medical College, New Scotland Avenue, Albany, NY 12208, USA
E-mail address: dubina@amc.edu

Phys Med Rehabil Clin N Am 29 (2018) 777–782
https://doi.org/10.1016/j.pmr.2018.06.011
1047-9651/18/© 2018 Elsevier Inc. All rights reserved.
pmr.theclinics.com

are uncomfortable discussing these issues with patients. Patient complaints may include pain with Valsalva-type activities, ambulation, prolonged sitting, prolonged standing, lumbar flexion, and/or extension. Patients may note these in isolation, combination, or in concert with complaints of urinary urgency, frequency, sensory dysesthesias in the perineum, and in males, erectile dysfunction.

DIFFERENTIAL DIAGNOSIS

The differential diagnosis of pelvic pain is rather broad-based, and encompasses primary pelvic pathology, bony pelvic issues, central as well as peripheral nervous system source generators, and lastly musculoskeletal pathology (**Table 1**).

PHYSICAL EXAMINATION

Securing a history and performance of a detailed physical examination, emphasizing the neuromusculoskeletal system are essential if one is to hope to elucidate what may be wrong, and where the problem may be. The time course of the problem should be noted. Factors that exacerbate as well as relieve the pain should be noted. Interventions and medication trials should be delved into, with questioning focusing on response or lack thereof to the intervention or medication trial.

A significant amount of information can be gleaned by observing the patient while taking a history. Note how the patient sits, stands, walks to the examining room, changes position from sit to stand, and moves about the examining room.

Work by Neville and Fitzgerald revealed that women with chronic pelvic pain were more likely to have abnormal musculoskeletal physical findings than pain-free women when tested by physical therapists on a subset of tests within a battery of examination maneuvers, including positive flexion, abduction, external rotation (FABER), forced FABER, hip scour test, posterior pelvic provocation test, and pelvic floor muscle tenderness noted on transrectal or transvaginal palpation.[2]

Work up for pelvic pain should include a detailed evaluation of the lumbosacral spine and observation of gait. A painful Trendelenburg gait pattern typically is secondary to true intra-articular hip joint dysfunction and presents with groin pain. A painless Trendelenburg gait pattern is commonly seen in disorders that result in weakness of the gluteus medius musculature. This may be secondary to underlying primary muscle disorders (myopathies) and should be considered when the findings are symmetric.

Table 1
Differential diagnosis considerations of pelvic pain

Musculoskeletal	Peripheral Nervous System	Central Nervous System	Primary Pelvic Pathology
Hip joint/labral pathology	Lumbosacral (L5, S1) radiculopathies	Central nervous system disorders	Primary pelvic pathology
Lumbosacral spine	Primary sacral radiculopathy secondary to Tarlov cysts	Multiple sclerosis	Pelvic floor dystonia-muscle overactivity/hypertonicity
Sacroiliac joint		Neuromyelitis optica	
Osteitis pubis	Isolated pudendal neuropathy (bicycle rider's neuropathy)	Cervical/thoracic myelopathy	Pelvic floor congestion syndrome
Ischial tuberosity bursitis		Spinal tumors-conus and cauda equina	Gynecologic pathology
	Peripheral neuropathy: toxic metabolic		s/p anal sphincter or prostate surgery
	Small fiber neuropathy		Postradiation therapy

Heel walking over distances may reveal subtle weakness of ankle dorsiflexors, and can help discern old L 5 radiculopathy with incomplete reinnervation as the etiology of a painless Trendelenburg gait that may become painful over long distances and result in cramping pelvic region discomfort because of muscle fatigue. Similarly, weakness of S1 innervated musculature can be brought out with long distance toe walking and may also explain deep gluteal pain with prolonged ambulation.

Reflexes may be normal, hypoactive, or hyperactive. Abnormal reflexes may provide useful insight into the etiology of the patient's symptoms. Hyporeflexia may be a manifestation of peripheral neuropathy, or polyradiculopathy secondary to lumbar spinal stenosis. Loss of Achilles reflexes is commonly seen in the previously mentioned scenarios; however, impaired sacral sensation is not typical in these situations. The combination of loss of an Achilles reflex in concert with impaired sacral sensation, especially if unilateral, can be observed in symptomatic sacral Tarlov cysts. Lower extremity hyperreflexia should raise the suspicion of thoracic or cervical myelopathy. In the case of cervical myelopathy, upper extremity hyperreflexia and altered sensation should be noted. Loss of a specific root level reflex in the upper extremities with hyperreflexia noted below the level of hyporeflexia is consistent with the diagnosis of cervical radiculomyelopathy. A cervical or thoracic radiculomyelopathy can result in pelvic pain either secondary to altered sensation as a result of an incomplete spinal cord or secondary to spasticity of pelvic floor musculature.

Physical examination of the hip should include an assessment of range of motion, looking for asymmetry of motion and pain with internal or external rotation. Groin pain with internal rotation is typical for internal derangement of the joint. Pain with external rotation may be labral in etiology but can also be seen in patients with iliotibial band/tensor fascia lata contracture, Intra-articular hip pathology will commonly manifest with complaints of groin pain and should always be considered in patients complaining of groin pain or deep lower quadrant pain. Persistent trochanteric region pain, despite treatment interventions, including physical therapy, modalities, and corticosteroid injection is a vexing problem and should raise suspicions. The complaint of poorly localized trochanteric region pain, and vague lateral hip discomfort can be the typically atypical presentation for an L 5 radiculopathy. Complicating this picture is the complaint of deep gluteal aching type discomfort, which may be described as pelvic pain. Altered gait mechanics can lead to pelvic pain, medial thigh pain, and pubic symphysis region pain. Lumbar spinal stenosis can present with complaints of low back pain and deep gluteal pain/pelvic pain. This is a not uncommon manifestation in patients with lower lumbar spinal stenosis that is central or neuroforaminal in etiology.

Several examination maneuvers can be useful in the assessment of pelvic pain patients. In all instances, the rationale for performing these test maneuvers is to try and localize the etiology of the pain. The forced FABER test allows the examiner to evaluate the role of the sacro iliac (SI) joint in the patient's complaint of pelvic pain. In the forced FABER test, the patient is placed in the supine position with one leg placed in FABER position. While maintained in this position, extra pressure is applied over the ipsilateral medial knee and contralateral ASIS. This results in a distracting force being placed thru the pelvis. The result of this test is stress placed thru the SI joint. A positive test is reproduction of pain in the SI. This test can also be performed in the seated position. Another test that has utility is the posterior pelvic pain provocation test. In this test the patient is maintained in a supine position. The hip is flexed to 90° on one side with a direct line force then applied thru the femur. This compresses the femoral-acetabular joint, resulting in transmission of a force vector through the ipsilateral SI joint. A positive test results in pain in the ipsilateral SI joint.[2]

Provocation of pelvic floor pain with palpation has also been shown to be a reproducible finding in women and men complaining of pelvic pain. In women, palpation of the pelvic floor can be carried out transvaginally with firm digital palpation to the right and left sides of the vaginal vault. Tension and trigger points in the pubococcygeus muscles can be noted on palpation. In males, surface palpation posterior to the scrotum to the right and left of midline has utility. The bulbocavernosus muscles are easily palpated in the male in this manner. One can assess symmetry of bulbocavernosus muscle bulk and sensitivity to palpation. In men and women, digital rectal examination will allow for palpation of the puborectalis and pubococcygeus muscles, as well as the deeper layers of the anal sphincter. A qualitative assessment of anal sphincter strength and endurance can also be ascertained during digital rectal examination.[2]

SPECIAL TESTS
MRI

Abnormalities noted on MRI scan may or may not correlate with the history and physical examination. Work by Silvis and colleagues[3] revealed a high prevalence of abnormal MRI findings in the pelvic, groin, and hip region in asymptomatic collegiate and professional hockey players. These included common adductor and or rectus abdominus muscle and tendon injuries with associated bone marrow edema in the symphysis pubis. Remarkably, partial and complete adductor or rectus abdominus tendon ruptures off the pubis were also noted in asymptomatic athletes. Hip abnormalities included acetabular labral tears and osteochondral lesions of the femoral head. MRI findings in the lumbar spine reveal a high prevalence of lumbar spine pathology in asymptomatic individuals.[4]

Work by Prather and colleagues[5] revealed in a retrospective review that 20% of patients with primary hip pathology had issues of refractory posterior pelvic pain as part of a symptom complex that also included groin pain and or lateral and anterior hip pain that was nonresponsive to conservative management. In this group of refractory posterior pelvic pain patients, 33% of them had complete resolution of their pain at 4.75 years after diagnostic and therapeutic hip arthroscopy. This would seem to indicate that in patients with early intra-articular hip pathology, including labral tears and early arthritis, posterior pelvic is a common clinical complaint.

Electrophysiologic Studies

EDX testing can have utility in the work up of the patient with pelvic pain. However, the test is not a stand-alone procedure, and the results need to be interpreted in the context of the historical data and examination findings., Additionally, there needs to be an appreciation of the limitations of the study and the unique nature of the musculature being studied.[2] For example, typical motor unit morphology noted on needle EMG of the anal sphincter is quite different when compared with more commonly studied skeletal muscle. Anal sphincter motor units are small amplitude (less than 500 uV), short duration (less than 8 ms), and polyphasic in morphology. In many respects, they look similar to classic myopathic motor units.[6,7]

Nerve Conduction Studies and Electrophysiologic Reflex Testing

Nerve conduction studies
Pudendal nerve conduction studies were originally described by Kiff and Swash in 1984.[8,9] These were used to investigate the possible link between pudendal neuropathy and stress urinary incontinence, as well as pelvic organ prolapse. Older patients and patients with an increased number of vaginal deliveries have been shown to have prolonged pudendal latencies using testing with St. Mark's electrodes.[10] Pudendal

nerve latencies have been used to predict outcome of anal sphincter repair with variable results. Chen and colleagues[11] reported positive outcomes from sphincter surgery even in patients with pudendal neuropathy. Conversely, Gilliland and colleagues[12] reported that bilateral normal pudendal nerve terminal motor latencies were the only factors predictive of long-term success following overlapping sphincteroplasty. Once again, appreciating that prolongation of latency by itself does not result in symptoms is key to understanding the confounding data that have been noted over the years regarding outcome from anal sphincter muscle repair.

Sacral reflex testing (penilo-cavernosus reflex, bulbocavernosus reflex, clitoro-anal reflex testing) can all be performed with EMG equipment. As in all instances of reflex arc testing, the absence of the reflex is what is of potential significance. A prolongation of the latency should not result in symptoms unless it is associated with partial or complete loss of axonal function (axonopathy vs conduction block). As such in all cases of latency prolongation, needle EMG of the anal sphincter/urethral sphincter or BC muscle should be performed. A clinically manifest clitoro-anal reflex may be difficult to obtain in women and can be absent in 20% of women with a normal neurologic examination. Given these findings, electrodiagnostic sacral reflex testing may have even greater utility in the work up of pelvic pain in females as opposed to males.[6]

Needle EMG

Needle EMG of sacral root innervated musculature (S2-4) can be performed to investigate pelvic pain complaints. Research by Podnar has demonstrated the utility of needle EMG of the external anal sphincter in concert with sacral reflex testing in the evaluation of a patient with cauda equina syndrome. The take home point on review of Podnar's data is that the combination of needle EMG and sacral reflex testing was more sensitive than either test by itself. More importantly, this study pointed out the critical nature of a detailed neurologic examination. Specific parameters identified as having high clinical yield and being highly correlative with electrophysiologic findings included anal sphincter squeeze, perianal sensation, and clinical penilo-cavernosus reflex. In fact, abnormalities in all 3 physical examination parameters correlated with electrophysiologic abnormalities in 96% of individuals with known cauda equina syndrome.[5]

The most sensitive stand-alone test for elucidating S2-4 root level pathology is needle EMG of either the anal or urethral sphincter. However, given the ease in which the anal sphincter can be accessed, it is the more practical of the 2 muscles to study.[5]

TREATMENT OF THE PROBLEM

Before the physician can hope to treat the patient's complaint of pelvic pain, the etiology of pain must first be identified. Once the driver of the pain is determined, treatment can be initiated.

Pelvic floor dysfunction of neurogenic etiology presents many challenges. Lower motor neuron lesions may result in pain and dysfunction from a combination of nerve injury and muscle weakness. Upper motor neuron lesions may result in pelvic pain from a combination of loss of neural control and increased muscle tone. Neuropathic pain of either UMN or LMN etiology presents an interesting constellation of dilemmas. Treatment ideally should be focused on treating the pain and the cause. Various therapies, including medications, prothrombin time (PT), and spinal cord stimulation may have utility in neuropathic pain management. More recent work by Rice, Albrecht, and colleagues, showed alterations in gene expression of CGRP in keratinocytes in patients with CRPS (personal communication). These findings raise interesting questions regarding mechanisms of nociceptive pain generation and its treatment.[13]

SUMMARY

The work up of pelvic pain can be challenging and rewarding. Securing the appropriate history and performing a detailed neurologic and musculoskeletal examination are critical. In patients with objective abnormal neurologic findings on examination, EMG testing can be helpful in localization of the pathology, delineating acuity versus chronicity, and potential for recovery.

Physiatrists should be asked to evaluate these patients on a more regular and routine basis. The training of physiatrists, with emphasis on evaluation of the neuro-musculoskeletal system, positions this field to be ideally suited as part of the team that will see and manage this complex group of patients.

REFERENCES

1. Zondervan KT, Yudkin PL, Vessey MP, et al. Chronic pelvic pain in the community - symptoms, investigations, and diagnoses. Am J Obstet Gynecol 2001;184: 1149–55.
2. Neville CE, Fitzgerald CM, Mallinson T, et al. A preliminary report of musculoskel-etal dysfunction in female chronic pelvic pain: a blinded study of examination findings. J Bodyw Mov Ther 2012;16(1):50–6.
3. Silvis ML, Mosher TJ, Smetana BS, et al. High prevalence of pelvic and hip mag-netic resonance imaging findings in asymmetric collegiate and professional hockey players. Am J Sports Med 2011;39(4):715–21.
4. Jensen MC, Brant-Zawadzki MN, Obuchowski N, et al. Magnetic resonance im-aging of the lumbar spine in people without back pain. N Engl J Med 1994; 331(2):69–73.
5. Prather H, Hunt D, Fournie A, et al. Early intra-articular hip disease presenting with posterior pelvic and groin pain. PM R 2009;1(9):809–15.
6. Podnar S. Sphincter electromyography and the penilo-cavernosus reflex: are both necessary? Neurourol Urodyn 2008;27:813–8.
7. Podnar S. Predictive value of the penilo-cavernosus reflex. Neurourol Urodyn 2009;28:390–4.
8. Kiff ES, SWash M. Normal proximal and delayed distal conduction in the puden-dal nerveof patients with idiopathic (neurogenic) faecal incontinence. J Neurol Neurosurg Psychiatr 1984;47:820–3.
9. Snooks SJ, Badenboch DF, Tiptaft RC, et al. Perineal nerve damage in genuine stress urinary incontinence. An electrophysiologic study. Br J Urol 1985;57: 422–6.
10. Olsen AI, Ross M, Stansfield RB, et al. Pelvic floor nerve conduction studies: es-tablishing clinically relevant normative data. Am J Obstet Gynecol 2003;189: 1114–9.
11. Chen AS, Luchtefeld MA, Senagore AJ, et al. Pudendal nerve latency. Does it predict outcome of anal sphincter surgery repair? Dis Colon Rectum 1998;41: 1005–9.
12. Gilliland R, Altomare DF, Moreira H Jr, et al. Pudendal neuropathy is predictive of failure following anterior overlapping sphincteroplasty. Dis Colon Rectum 1998; 41:1516–22.
13. Hou Q, Barr T, Gee L, et al. Keratinocyte expression of calcitonin gene-related peptide β: implications for neuropathic and inflammatory pain mechanisms. Pain 2011;152(9):2036–51.

Guiding Treatment for Foot Pain

David Del Toro, MD*, P. Andrew Nelson, MD

KEYWORDS

- Tibial nerve • Peroneal nerve • Electrodiagnostic • EDX • Tarsal tunnel syndrome
- Foot pain

KEY POINTS

- In the electrodiagnostic approach of the patient who presents with foot pain, numbness, and/or tingling, it is important to consider a broad differential diagnosis of both neuropathic and nonneuropathic conditions, including focal and systemic causes.
- A vital precursor to this type of electrophysiologic study is that one needs to have a firm understanding of the neuroanatomy of the foot and ankle, with a particular focus on the local neuroanatomy, including potential entrapment sites.
- The electrodiagnostic evaluation of the foot typically requires numerous motor and sensory nerve conduction studies, as well as needle electromyography examination of various intrinsic foot muscles.
- A well conceived and organized electrodiagnostic assessment incorporating a combination of the most appropriate NCS and needle EMG of relevant intrinsic foot muscles can localize a neurogenic pathology and guide appropriate treatment of a patient with foot pain.

INTRODUCTION

In the electrodiagnostic (EDX) approach of the patient who presents with foot pain, numbness, and/or tingling, it is important to consider a broad differential diagnosis of both neuropathic and nonneuropathic conditions, including focal and systemic causes. A vital precursor to this type of electrophysiologic study is that one needs to have a firm understanding of the neuroanatomy of the foot and ankle with a particular focus on the local neuroanatomy, including potential entrapment sites. The EDX evaluation of the foot typically requires numerous motor and sensory nerve conduction studies (NCS) as well as needle electromyography (EMG) examination of various intrinsic foot muscles. This article assists the electromyographer in the selection and utilization of the most appropriate EDX studies, both NCS and needle EMG

Disclosure: The authors have nothing to disclose.
Department of Physical Medicine and Rehabilitation, Medical College of Wisconsin, 8701 Watertown Plank Road, Milwaukee, WI 53226, USA
* Corresponding author.
E-mail address: ddeltoro@mcw.edu

Phys Med Rehabil Clin N Am 29 (2018) 783–792
https://doi.org/10.1016/j.pmr.2018.06.012
1047-9651/18/© 2018 Elsevier Inc. All rights reserved.

pmr.theclinics.com

examination, for evaluation. The EDX findings and impression can then help guide potential treatment options for the patient with foot pain and other symptoms. Moreover, this discussion demonstrates the added value that EDX evaluation of the foot provides to the comprehensive assessment of foot pain.

ANATOMY
Fibular (Peroneal) Nerve

The common fibular nerve (CFN, also known as the common peroneal nerve) branches from the sciatic nerve proximal to the knee and descends in the posterolateral knee and around the fibular head, where it then divides into the superficial fibular nerve (SFN) and the deep fibular nerve (DFN). Both branches contain fibers originating from the L5 and S1 nerve roots.

The SFN innervates the fibularis longus and brevis in the lateral compartment of the leg and then enters the foot at the anterolateral ankle (superficial to the inferior extensor retinaculum) and supplies cutaneous innervation to the dorsal ankle and foot. In approximately 28% of cases, the SFN supplies an accessory branch of the DFN that travels posterior to the lateral malleolus and then innervates the extensor digitorum brevis (EDB).[1]

The DFN courses through the anterior compartment of the leg (where it supplies motor innervation) before dividing into medial and lateral branches just proximal to the ankle. Both branches then pass deep to the inferior extensor retinaculum (sometimes referred to as the anterior tarsal tunnel).[2] The lateral branch provides motor innervation to the EDB. The medial branch supplies cutaneous innervation to the first dorsal web space. In 92.1% of cases, the medial branch also supplies some motor innervation to the first dorsal interosseous pedis (DIP), with significantly less innervation to the second and third dorsal interossei.[3]

Tibial Nerve

The tibial nerve (TN), carrying fibers from the S1 and S2 nerve roots, enters the foot posterior to the medial malleolus deep to the overlying flexor retinaculum within the tarsal tunnel. In the upper, or proximal, tarsal tunnel there is a distinct compartment for the TN, which is a potential site of entrapment.[3] The TN has 4 terminal branches: the medial plantar nerve (MPN), lateral plantar nerve (LPN), first branch of the LPN (also referred to as inferior calcaneal nerve or Baxter's nerve), and the medial calcaneal nerve[4] (**Fig. 1**).

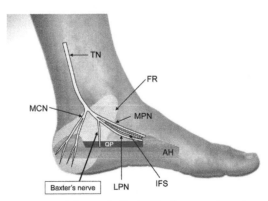

Fig. 1. The tibial nerve. AH, abductor hallucis; FR, flexor retinaculum; IFS, interfascicular septum; QP, quadratus plantae; TN, tibial nerve. (Copyright AANEM, Nandedkar Productions, LLC, 2008.)

The medial calcaneal nerve (MCN) branches from the TN variably from within, proximal or distal to the tarsal tunnel. It is typically a purely sensory nerve and supplies sensation to the medial, posterior, and plantar heel.[5]

In 93% to 95% of cases, the TN divides into the MPN and LPN within the tarsal tunnel. The lower, or distal, tarsal tunnel is divided into upper and lower calcaneal chambers, which are separated by the interfascicular septum. The MPN travels within the upper chamber, whereas the lower chamber contains the LPN. Both chambers can be a site of possible entrapment for its specific plantar branch.[3]

After exiting the upper calcaneal chamber, the MPN travels through the abductor canal, a known entrapment site of the MPN, into the medial sole of the foot. The MPN innervates the abductor hallucis (AH), medial and lateral heads of the flexor hallucis brevis, flexor digitorum brevis (FDB), and the first lumbrical. It provides sensation to the medial sole of the foot, the plantar surface of the first to third toes, and the medial half of the fourth toe.[3,6]

The LPN leaves the lower calcaneal chamber and courses into the sole of the foot through its own abductor canal, a potential site of entrapment for this nerve. It then passes laterally and distally across the foot and divides into its terminal superficial and deep branches. The LPN supplies motor innervation to the quadratus plantae (QP), adductor hallucis, flexor digiti minimi brevis, lateral head of flexor hallucis brevis, all interossei, and second to fourth lumbricals. Sensory innervation is supplied to the lateral sole of the foot, plantar surface of the fifth toe and lateral half of the fourth toe.[3,6]

In the upper tarsal tunnel, the first branch of the LPN (or Baxter's nerve) can arise from the LPN directly, as a trifurcation of the TN or just proximal to the bifurcation of the MPN and LPN (directly off the TN). It enters the lower calcaneal chamber but then penetrates the posterior chamber and travels between the AH and QP in the medial heel, which is a possible site of compression. It then courses laterally, and just anterior to the medial aspect of the calcaneal tuberosity, between QP and FDB.[3] The nerve can be compressed by a heel spur at the medial calcaneal tuberosity or involved in chronic plantar fasciitis[7] at the same site. The first branch of the LPN always terminates with motor innervation to the abductor digiti minimi pedis (also known as abductor digiti quinti pedis); it can also give motor branches to QP and FDB. In addition, the first branch of the LPN supplies periosteal afferent branches to the calcaneus but not cutaneous, innervation.[4]

Sural Nerve

In the popliteal fossa the sciatic nerve divides into the TN and fibular nerve. The TN gives rise to the medial sural cutaneous nerve in the popliteal fossa. In the mid-calf it is joined by a communicating branch from the CFN (lateral sural cutaneous nerve) to form the sural nerve.[8] The sural nerve supplies sensation to the lateral ankle and heel, as well as the lateral foot. It does not provide any motor innervation.

Saphenous Nerve

The saphenous nerve is a cutaneous branch of the femoral nerve that originates in the thigh. Below the knee it descends along the medial tibial border and enters the foot at the anteromedial ankle and supplies sensation to the proximal medial dorsum of the foot; it does not provide motor innervation.

NEUROGENIC CONDITIONS AFFECTING THE FOOT
Tibial Neuropathy

Tarsal tunnel syndrome (TTS) is defined as a focal compressive neuropathy of the posterior TN because it passes behind the medial malleolus under the overlying flexor retinaculum. The clinical presentation can vary depending on the terminal branch affected but typically involves numbness, tingling, burning, cramping, or painful paresthesias in the sole of the foot (medial and lateral aspect), plantar heel, and plantar surface of the toes. Symptoms may be aggravated with prolonged standing or ambulation. Weakness is not commonly noted by patients but in severe cases focal intrinsic foot muscle atrophy can be observed.[3] Tinel sign over the TN may be positive. Sensory deficit usually is noted in the sole of the foot, plantar aspect of the toes, and plantar heel.[9] TTS can be caused by space occupying or compressive lesions; trauma; postsurgical, biomechanical traction on the nerve; systemic diseases such as rheumatoid arthritis or diabetes mellitus; or edema. Needle EMG examination is crucial in determining which TN branches are affected.

The MPN may be compressed in its abductor canal between the abductor hallucis and its attachment to the talus and navicular bone. MPN mononeuropathy is sometimes referred to as "jogger's foot" and may be seen in patients with hindfoot valgus and pes planus. Patients often report exercise-induced pain on the medial plantar surface of the foot, often radiating distally to the plantar surface of the first, second, and third toes (and possibly the medial half of the fourth toe).[3,10] Dysesthesias or numbness may be present along the medial heel, arch, and medial sole of the foot and the first through third toes.

The LPN enters the sole of the foot through its own abductor canal, formed by the attachment of the abductor hallucis to the talus and navicular bone, which is a potential site of entrapment for the LPN. Symptoms of involvement of the LPN can include pain or paresthesias affecting the lateral plantar surface of the foot extending to the plantar fifth toe and lateral half of the fourth toe.[3]

The MCN can branch from the TN proximal to, within, or distal to the tarsal tunnel. A compressive lesion affecting the MCN can result in pain and paresthesias in the medial heel and sensation may be reduced in medial, posterior, and plantar heel. There is typically no motor involvement as it is usually a purely sensory nerve.[5]

The first branch of the LPN (or Baxter's nerve) may be entrapped between the AH and the medial edge of QP, where it is susceptible due to hyperpronation. Another location of potential compression is between the FDB and the medial calcaneal tuberosity or due to a bone spur from the medial calcaneus. Patients often complain of medial plantar heel pain similar to that of plantar fasciitis. In contrast to plantar fasciitis, symptoms representative of a first branch lateral plantar neuropathy are more medial and proximal and tend to worsen with activity. Pain can radiate to the medial ankle or laterally across the proximal plantar foot. Paresthesias and weakness are not typically reported, but clinical examination may reveal inability to abduct the fifth toe.[3,11,12]

Fibular Neuropathy

The DFN can be entrapped under the inferior extensor retinaculum, often referred to as anterior TTS. Tight or rigid footwear may cause compression of the DFN and the nerve can be injured by local trauma. The lateral and/or medial branches of the DFN may be affected. If the lateral branch is affected, it may result in pain across the dorsal foot and ankle. Weakness may not be noted by the patient but if severely involved, atrophy of

EDB may be present. Paresthesias may be noted in the first dorsal web space with involvement of the medial branch.[2,8] In addition, the medial branch commonly sends motor fibers to the first DIP and with much less frequency to second and third DIP.[3]

The SFN can be injured due to a laceration or trauma anywhere along its course but is most commonly entrapped because it pierces the deep fascia 10 to 12 cm proximal to the anterior ankle. It may also be injured in an inversion ankle sprain or functional ankle instability due to a traction injury to the nerve. Symptoms often involve pain and paresthesias in the dorsal ankle and foot, typically sparing the first dorsal web space and plantar foot. There is no motor involvement because distally the SFN supplies only sensory innervation.[8,13]

The most frequent fibular neuropathy is compression of the CFN at the fibular head. This can occur due to sitting with crossed legs, rapid weight loss or wasting of the leg musculature (particularly in the setting of prolonged bed rest), prolonged squatting, or other external compression or stretch of the nerve. Proximal fibular fracture or nerve injury associated with surgical positioning, knee arthroscopy, or arthroplasty may also result in CFN injury.[8,14] Both the superficial and the deep branches can be affected resulting in ankle dorsiflexor weakness (foot drop) and variable pain or paresthesias in the distal lateral leg and dorsum of the foot and ankle.

Sural Neuropathy

Isolated sural neuropathies are rare but can occur due to local trauma, fractures, ganglia, or compression by fibrotic bands or tight boots. The most common entrapment sites are along the lateral border of the ankle, the calcaneus, and the fifth metatarsal. In addition, sural neuropathy is often secondary to ankle surgery and the subsequent scarring, bony hypertrophy, or instability. The sural nerve may also be injured during ankle arthroscopic surgery. Pain or paresthesias in the lateral ankle and heel to the lateral foot are common symptoms.[15,16] There is no motor innervation, thus any associated ankle weakness should raise the suspicion of a more proximal neurogenic lesion, a different peripheral nerve injury, or more diffuse neurogenic process.

Saphenous Neuropathy

Entrapment of the saphenous nerve is rare at the ankle or foot, typically occurring more proximally. Distal compression is often secondary to trauma or surgery. Patients present with pain or paresthesias in the anterior and medial ankle and foot.

Morton Neuroma

Morton neuroma is a focal neuropathy of the interdigital nerve near the distal edge of the intermetatarsal ligament. It occurs most commonly in the third intermetatarsal space (between the third and fourth toes) and occasionally in the second or fourth web space. The neuroma consists primarily of perineural fibrosis and degenerative changes. Patients typically complain of burning or electrical pain in the web space and sometimes paresthesias. Symptoms frequently worsen with physical activity and can be reproduced with direct palpation.[9] EDX studies are normal but can rule out more proximal tibial (or terminal branch) lesions and lumbosacral radiculopathy.

Lumbosacral Radiculopathy

Lumbosacral radiculopathy involving the L5 or S1 nerve roots is a common disorder and can be a potential source of foot symptoms. As in distal ankle and foot entrapment neuropathies, radiculopathies are typically unilateral. Sensory NCS are typically normal as most causes of radiculopathy occur proximal to the dorsal root ganglion. A significant degree of axonal loss of the L5, S1, or S2 nerve roots must occur before compound muscle action potential amplitudes in motor NCS demonstrate abnormalities, typically occurring only in advanced cases of radiculopathy. Needle EMG examination is more sensitive for axonal loss than NCS. In addition to intrinsic foot muscles, proximal leg muscles with L5 and S1 innervation as well as lumbar paraspinals should be examined. A radiculopathy is implied with EMG abnormalities in 2 or more muscles with different peripheral nerve supply but the same nerve root involvement, including the lumbar paraspinals. In addition, needle EMG findings should be normal in adjacent myotomes.[8]

Peripheral Neuropathy

The most common pattern of peripheral neuropathy is a distal, symmetric length-dependent process resulting initially in bilateral foot symptoms. The pattern of NCS findings can help determine if the process is primarily axonal or demyelinating in nature, which can assist in narrowing the differential diagnosis. Sensory and motor NCS can show prolonged latencies, decreased conduction velocity, and reduced amplitudes in multiple peripheral nerves. In addition, in an axonal process, needle EMG findings would typically reveal abnormal spontaneous activity and possibly motor unit action potential morphology changes in distal foot and leg muscles but not more proximal leg muscles with similar nerve root innervation.[8]

NONNEUROGENIC CAUSES OF FOOT PAIN

There are numerous nonneuropathic causes of foot and ankle pain that can mimic neuropathic conditions and should be considered in the differential diagnosis. A careful history and physical examination can typically assist in narrowing the cause of the symptoms. Nonneuropathic causes do not tend to cause paresthesias or sensory loss. Although not always necessary to make a diagnosis, EDX studies would be expected to be normal in these conditions.

Plantar fasciitis is a common overuse condition of the plantar fascia at its attachment to the calcaneus. Heel pain is a primary complaint, often worse in the morning and with initial steps but improves during the day. Point tenderness at the medial calcaneal tuberosity may extend along the medial border of the plantar fascia and stretching the fascia may reproduce pain. Plantar heel pain can be due to fat pad contusion (or atrophy) due to excessive heel strike. Calcaneal stress fracture can result from marching or running, typically insidious in onset. Tenderness can be present over the medial or lateral calcaneus, and pain can be reproduced by squeezing the calcaneus.[17]

The Achilles tendon inserts at the posterior calcaneus and is a common cause of posterior heel pain. Achilles tendinopathy is an overuse tendon injury, although partial or complete tears can also occur. Achilles regional pain often develops gradually with pain and stiffness on waking that can improve with walking. Retrocalcaneal bursitis is another common cause of posterior heel pain as the retrocalcaneal bursa lies between the posterior aspect of the calcaneus and the insertion of the Achilles tendon and can become inflamed.[17]

Ankle sprains most commonly result from inversion injuries rather than eversion due to the relative weakness of the lateral ligaments compared with the medial ligament. The most common site of pain is over the anterolateral ankle involving the anterior talofibular ligament. Pain is often focal and provoked with weight bearing, palpation, and

Table 1		
NCS in EDX evaluation of the foot		
Motor	**Sensory**	**Mixed**
MPN	MPN	MPN
LPN	LPN	LPN
First branch of LPN (aka Baxter's nerve)	Superficial fibular	
Deep fibular	Deep fibular	
	Sural	
	Medial calcaneal	
	Saphenous	

passive ankle movements depending on the involved structures. There can also be local swelling and bruising in more severe injuries.

Medial ankle pain can occur in the absence of an acute injury due to overuse and excessive pronation. Tibialis posterior (TP) tendinopathy or flexor hallucis tendinopathy can result in pain posterior to the medial malleolus and may radiate along the line of the TP tendon to its insertion on the navicular or into the medial arch of the foot. The absence of sensory symptoms can assist in distinguishing a tendinopathy from TTS or a tibial branch neuropathy.

ELECTRODIAGNOSTIC EVALUATION OF THE FOOT
Nerve Conduction Studies

NCS, which are available and feasible to be used in EDX evaluation of the patient presenting with foot symptoms (pain, numbness, and/or tingling) would include motor NCS along with sensory and mixed NCS. Most of these NCS techniques are routine studies that can be found in standard NCS manuals.[18,19] The motor NCS include 3 TN branches (MPN, LPN, and first branch of LPN) and the DFN. The sensory NCS consist of MPN, LPN, superficial fibular, deep fibular, sural, medial calcaneal, and saphenous nerves while the mixed NCS are composed of MPN and LPN. It is the author's experience that due to the time commitment necessary to perform sensory NCS of the MPN and LPN (averaging >100 stimuli) and the relatively small amplitude of the averaged response that is recorded (2–5 μV), these sensory NCS can be challenging and therefore, diagnostic utility may be of limited value (**Table 1**).

Needle Electromyography Examination

Along with NCS, the needle EMG examination is a vital and necessary part of the EDX evaluation of any patient presenting with foot pain, numbness, and/or tingling. Moreover, in the author's clinical experience due to the subtle nature of the electrophysiologic findings and pathophysiology associated with entrapment neuropathies in the foot, the needle EMG examination of intrinsic foot muscles may likely be more sensitive than the motor and sensory NCS. To evaluate specific TN branches and the DFN, multiple intrinsic foot muscles can be studied during the needle EMG examination. The intrinsic foot muscles include abductor hallucis, first DIP, fourth DIP, EDB, abductor digiti minimi (or quinti) pedis and flexor digiti minimi brevis. The peripheral nerve innervation pattern of these intrinsic foot muscles is outlined later in this article (**Table 2**).

GUIDE TO TREATMENT BASED ON ELECTRODIAGNOSTIC IMPRESSION

After meticulous clinical evaluation of the patient's lower extremities with particular focus on the foot, careful selection of the pertinent NCS from those listed

Table 2
Peripheral nerve innervation of intrinsic foot muscles

Intrinsic Foot Muscles	Peripheral Nerve Innervation
Abductor hallucis	MPN
First DIP	Deep fibular nerve + LPN
Fourth DIP	LPN
Extensor digitorum brevis	Deep fibular nerve
Abductor digiti minimi (or quinti) pedis	First branch of LPN (aka Baxter's nerve)
Flexor digiti minimi brevis	LPN

earlier (See **Table 1**) along with needle EMG examination of the lower extremity, including the relevant intrinsic foot muscles, should provide a comprehensive EDX evaluation of the foot. Armed with a well conceived and organized EDX approach that incorporates a combination of the abovementioned NCS and needle EMG examination of appropriate intrinsic foot muscles, this electrophysiologic assessment can guide suitable treatment for the patient with foot pain or other symptoms.

For example, after undergoing the appropriate EDX evaluation, the patient with a potential entrapment neuropathy in the foot involving the MPN, it is likely this patient would undergo advanced imaging (ultrasound or MRI) to evaluate for a space-occupying mass or potential scar tissue or fibrosis (if there is a history of trauma or relevant surgery). If this were negative, then the patient may have a trial of conservative management such as being fitted with a custom orthotic. **Table 3** indicates how the EDX impression can guide further evaluation and potential treatment options. However, this is not meant to be a comprehensive list of evaluation techniques or treatment measures but simply a "road map" to give the electromyographer some direction.

Table 3
Treatment guide based on electrodiagnostic impression

EDX Impression	Further Evaluation	Potential Treatment Options
Entrapment neuropathy in the foot (MPN, LPN, first branch of LPN, or fibular nerve)	Advanced imaging (US or MRI)	• Custom orthotic • Other conservative measures • Surgery (if indicated)
Peripheral polyneuropathy	Laboratory workup for cause	• Neuromodulating medications, custom orthotics, physical therapy
L5-S1 radiculopathy	Advanced imaging (MRI)	• Physical therapy • Neuromodulator medications, antiinflammatories • Possible epidural steroid injection • Surgery (if indicated)
Nonneuropathic causes (plantar fasciitis, Achilles tendinopathy, ankle sprain)	Advanced imaging (if needed)	• Typical soft tissue injury or MSK-oriented conservative measures (PT, orthotics, etc)

Abbreviations: MSK, musculoskeletal; PT, physical therapy; US, ultrasound.

SUMMARY

In the evaluation of a patient presenting with foot pain, numbness, and/or tingling, EDX studies can be invaluable in determining the cause and directing subsequent evaluation and treatment. A solid knowledge of foot and ankle anatomy, with an emphasis on neuroanatomy, is fundamental for establishing a differential diagnosis and organizing a thoughtful EDX approach. Needle EMG examination of selected intrinsic foot muscles is an integral part in the EDX evaluation of the foot and can be more sensitive than motor and sensory NCS, particularly for entrapment neuropathies in the foot such as TTS. The history and physical examination, NCS, and needle EMG examination must all correlate and fit to arrive at a correct impression that is logical anatomically and physiologically.

REFERENCES

1. Park TA, Del Toro DR. Electrodiagnostic evaluation of the foot. Phys Med Rehabil Clin N Am 1998;9(4):871–96.
2. Park TA, Del Toro DR. Isolated inferior calcaneal neuropathy. Muscle Nerve 1996; 19(1):106–8.
3. Park TA, Del Toro DR. The medial calcaneal nerve: anatomy and nerve conduction technique. Muscle Nerve 1995;18(1):32–8.
4. Ngo KT, Del Toro DR. Electrodiagnostic findings and surgical outcome in isolated first branch lateral plantar neuropathy: a case series with literature review. Arch Phys Med Rehabil 2010;91(12):1948–51.
5. Chundru U, Liebeskind A, Seidelmann F, et al. Plantar fasciitis and calcaneal spur formation are associated with abductor digiti minimi atrophy on MRI of the foot. Skeletal Radiol 2008;37(6):505–10.
6. Roy PC. Electrodiagnostic evaluation of lower extremity neurogenic problems. Foot Ankle Clin N Am 2011;16:225–42.
7. Blackshear BM, Lutz GE, Obrien SJ. Sural nerve entrapment after injury to the gastrocnemius: a case report. Arch Phys Med Rehabil 1999;80:604–5.
8. Asp JP, Rand JA. Peroneal nerve palsy after total knee arthroplasty. Clin Orthop Relat Res 1990;261:233–7.
9. Gesini L, Jandolo B, Pietrangeli A. The anterior tarsal tunnel syndrome. J Bone Joint Surg Am 1984;66:786–7.
10. Gutmann L. Atypical deep peroneal neuropathy in the presence of accessory deep peroneal nerve. J Neurol Neurosurg Psychiatry 1970;33:453–6.
11. Havel PE, Ebraheim NA, Clark SE, et al. Tibial branching in the tarsal tunnel. Foot Ankle 1988;9:117–9.
12. Pomeroy G, Wilton J, Anthony S. Entrapment neuropathy about the foot and ankle: an update. J Am Acad Orthop Surg 2015;23:58–66.
13. Bregman PJ, Schuenke M. Current diagnosis and treatment of superficial fibular nerve injuries and entrapment. Clin Podiatr Med Surg 2016;33:243–54.
14. Stickler DE, Morley KN, Massey EW. Sural neuropathy: etiologies and predisposing factors. Muscle Nerve 2006;34:482–4.
15. Flanigan RM, DiGiovanni BF. Peripheral nerve entrapments of the lower leg, ankle, and foot. Foot Ankle Clin N Am 2011;16:255–74.
16. Sarrafian SK. Anatomy of the foot and ankle. Philadelphia: JB Lippincott Company; 1983.
17. Brukner P, Khan K. Clinical sports medicine. 4th edition. New York: McGraw-Hill Medical; 2011.

18. Buschbacher RM, Kumbhare DA, Robinson LR. Buschbacher's manual of nerve conduction studies. 3rd edition. New York: Demos Medical; 2016.

19. DeLisa JA, Mackenzie K, Baran EM. Manual of nerve conduction velocity and somatosensory evoked potentials. 2nd edition. New York: Raven Press Books; 1987.

UNITED STATES POSTAL SERVICE ® Statement of Ownership, Management, and Circulation (All Periodicals Publications Except Requester Publications)

1. Publication Title	2. Publication Number	3. Filing Date
PHYSICAL MEDICINE AND REHABILITATION CLINICS OF NORTH AMERICA	009 – 243	9/18/2018

4. Issue Frequency	5. Number of Issues Published Annually	6. Annual Subscription Price
FEB, MAY, AUG, NOV	4	$294.00

7. Complete Mailing Address of Known Office of Publication (Not printer) (Street, city, county, state, and ZIP+4®)

ELSEVIER INC.
230 Park Avenue, Suite 800
New York, NY 10169

Contact Person
STEPHEN R. BUSHING

Telephone (Include area code)
215-239-3688

8. Complete Mailing Address of Headquarters or General Business Office of Publisher (Not printer)

ELSEVIER INC.
230 Park Avenue, Suite 800
New York, NY 10169

9. Full Names and Complete Mailing Addresses of Publisher, Editor, and Managing Editor (Do not leave blank)

Publisher (Name and complete mailing address)

TAYLOR E. BALL, ELSEVIER INC.
1600 JOHN F KENNEDY BLVD. SUITE 1800
PHILADELPHIA, PA 19103-2899

Editor (Name and complete mailing address)

LAUREN BOYLE, ELSEVIER INC.
1600 JOHN F KENNEDY BLVD. SUITE 1800
PHILADELPHIA, PA 19103-2899

Managing Editor (Name and complete mailing address)

PATRICK MANLEY, ELSEVIER INC.
1600 JOHN F KENNEDY BLVD. SUITE 1800
PHILADELPHIA, PA 19103-2899

10. Owner (Do not leave blank. If the publication is owned by a corporation, give the name and address of the corporation immediately followed by the names and addresses of all stockholders owning or holding 1 percent or more of the total amount of stock. If not owned by a corporation, give the names and addresses of the individual owners. If owned by a partnership or other unincorporated firm, give its name and address as well as those of each individual owner. If the publication is published by a nonprofit organization, give its name and address.)

Full Name	Complete Mailing Address
WHOLLY OWNED SUBSIDIARY OF REED/ELSEVIER, US HOLDINGS	1600 JOHN F KENNEDY BLVD. SUITE 1800 PHILADELPHIA, PA 19103-2899

11. Known Bondholders, Mortgagees, and Other Security Holders Owning or Holding 1 Percent or More of Total Amount of Bonds, Mortgages, or Other Securities. If none, check box ▶ ☐ None

Full Name	Complete Mailing Address
N/A	

12. Tax Status (For completion by nonprofit organizations authorized to mail at nonprofit rates) (Check one)
The purpose, function, and nonprofit status of this organization and the exempt status for federal income tax purposes:
☒ Has Not Changed During Preceding 12 Months
☐ Has Changed During Preceding 12 Months (Publisher must submit explanation of change with this statement)

PS Form **3526**, July 2014 [Page 1 of 4 (see instructions page 4)] PSN: 7530-01-000-9931 PRIVACY NOTICE: See our privacy policy on www.usps.com

13. Publication Title				14. Issue Date for Circulation Data Below	
PHYSICAL MEDICINE AND REHABILITATION CLINICS OF NORTH AMERICA				MAY 2018	
15. Extent and Nature of Circulation				Average No. Copies Each Issue During Preceding 12 Months	No. Copies of Single Issue Published Nearest to Filing Date
a. Total Number of Copies (Net press run)				173	265
b. Paid Circulation (By Mail and Outside the Mail)	(1)	Mailed Outside-County Paid Subscriptions Stated on PS Form 3541 (Include paid distribution above nominal rate, advertiser's proof copies, and exchange copies)		83	126
	(2)	Mailed In-County Paid Subscriptions Stated on PS Form 3541 (Include paid distribution above nominal rate, advertiser's proof copies, and exchange copies)		0	0
	(3)	Paid Distribution Outside the Mails Including Sales Through Dealers and Carriers, Street Vendors, Counter Sales, and Other Paid Distribution Outside USPS®		36	53
	(4)	Paid Distribution by Other Classes of Mail Through the USPS (e.g., First-Class Mail®)		0	0
c. Total Paid Distribution (Sum of 15b (1), (2), (3), and (4))			▶	119	179
d. Free or Nominal Rate Distribution (By Mail and Outside the Mail)	(1)	Free or Nominal Rate Outside-County Copies included on PS Form 3541		44	68
	(2)	Free or Nominal Rate In-County Copies Included on PS Form 3541		0	0
	(3)	Free or Nominal Rate Copies Mailed at Other Classes Through the USPS (e.g., First-Class Mail)		0	0
	(4)	Free or Nominal Rate Distribution Outside the Mail (Carriers or other means)		0	0
e. Total Free or Nominal Rate Distribution (Sum of 15d (1), (2), (3) and (4))			▶	44	68
f. Total Distribution (Sum of 15c and 15e)			▶	163	247
g. Copies not Distributed (See Instructions to Publishers #4 (page 63))			▶	10	18
h. Total (Sum of 15f and g)			▶	173	265
i. Percent Paid (15c divided by 15f times 100)			▶	73.01%	72.47%

* If you are claiming electronic copies, go to line 16 on page 3. If you are not claiming electronic copies, skip to line 17 on page 3.

16. Electronic Copy Circulation		Average No. Copies Each Issue During Preceding 12 Months	No. Copies of Single Issue Published Nearest to Filing Date
a. Paid Electronic Copies	▶	0	0
b. Total Paid Print Copies (Line 15c) + Paid Electronic Copies (Line 16a)	▶	119	179
c. Total Print Distribution (Line 15f) + Paid Electronic Copies (Line 16a)	▶	163	247
d. Percent Paid (Both Print & Electronic Copies) (16b divided by 16c × 100)	▶	73.01%	72.47%

☒ I certify that 50% of all my distributed copies (electronic and print) are paid above a nominal price.

17. Publication of Statement of Ownership

☒ If the publication is a general publication, publication of this statement is required. Will be printed in the **NOVEMBER 2018** issue of this publication. ☐ Publication not required.

18. Signature and Title of Editor, Publisher, Business Manager, or Owner

STEPHEN R. BUSHING - INVENTORY DISTRIBUTION CONTROL MANAGER

Stephen R. Bushing   Date 9/18/2018

I certify that all information furnished on this form is true and complete. I understand that anyone who furnishes false or misleading information on this form or who omits material or information requested on the form may be subject to criminal sanctions (including fines and imprisonment) and/or civil sanctions (including civil penalties).

PS Form **3526**, July 2014 (Page 3 of 4) PRIVACY NOTICE: See our privacy policy on www.usps.com

Moving?

Make sure your subscription moves with you!

To notify us of your new address, find your **Clinics Account Number** (located on your mailing label above your name), and contact customer service at:

Email: journalscustomerservice-usa@elsevier.com

800-654-2452 (subscribers in the U.S. & Canada)
314-447-8871 (subscribers outside of the U.S. & Canada)

Fax number: 314-447-8029

Elsevier Health Sciences Division
Subscription Customer Service
3251 Riverport Lane
Maryland Heights, MO 63043

*To ensure uninterrupted delivery of your subscription, please notify us at least 4 weeks in advance of move.

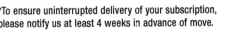